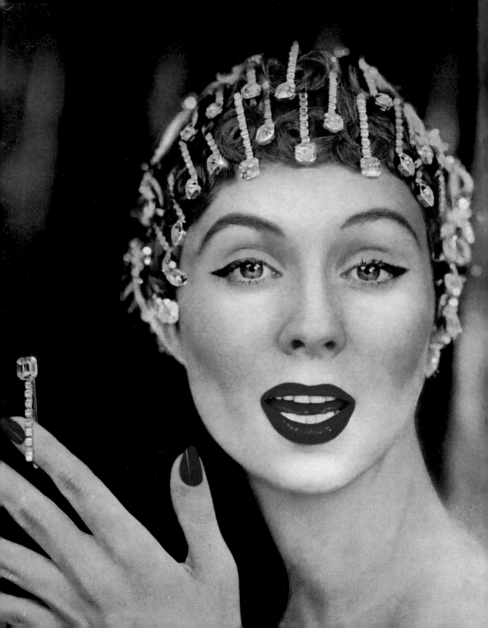

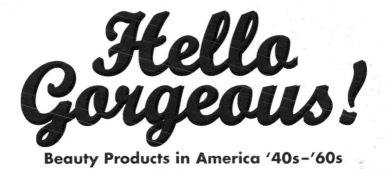

Hello Gorgeous!

Beauty Products in America '40s–'60s

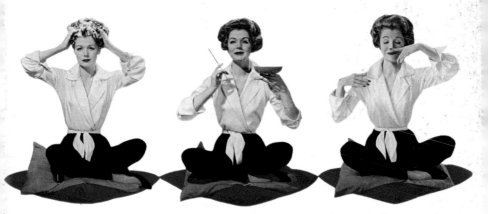

Rachel C. Weingarten

PORTLAND, OREGON

Cover Design: Kevin A. Welsch, Collectors Press, Inc.
Book Design: Kevin A. Welsch, James Fletcher, Ryan Crews, Collectors Press, Inc.
Editors: Lindsay Brown, Julie Steigerwaldt, and Jennifer Weaver-Neist
Proofreader: Ali McCart

Library of Congress Cataloging-in-Publication Data

Weingarten, Rachel C.
  Hello, gorgeous! : beauty products in America, 40s-60s / by Rachel C. Weingarten.-- 1st American ed.
    p.   cm.
  ISBN 1-933112-18-2 (pbk. : alk. paper)
  1. Beauty culture--United States--History--20th century. 2. Beauty, Personal--United States--History--20th century. 3. Cosmetics--United States--History--20th century. I. Title.

GT499.W43 2006
646.7'2--dc22

                    2005032746

Distributed by Publishers Group West

First American Edition
    ISBN 1-933112-18-2

Printed in China
9 8 7 6 5 4 3 2 1

Collectors Press books are available at special discounts for bulk purchases, premiums, and promotions. Special editions, including personalized inserts or covers, and corporate logos, can be printed in quantity for special purposes. For further information contact: Special sales, Collectors Press, Inc., P.O. Box 230986, Portland, OR 97281. Toll free: 1.800.423.1848.

For a free catalog: Toll Free 1.800.423.1848 or visit collectorspress.com.

Contents

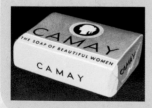

Introduction
◇◇◇◆◇ ▣ ◇◆◇◇◇

Sex sells. Beauty seduces. Classic beauty advertising both sells and seduces. The beauty advertisements of the 1940s, 1950s, and 1960s convinced women to buy beauty products to help them seduce men. These ads promised "miraculous" new formulations, "scientific" innovations, and "thrilling" results. In other words, beauty advertising of the mid-twentieth century wasn't all that different from today.

To put things into historical perspective, the era before World War II was marked with intense privation culminating in the Great Depression. The Greatest Generation barely had time to catch its collective breath after this devastation before being plunged into war.

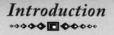

Brave GIs fought overseas, while their previously pampered counterparts worked in factories to keep the war effort going. The music of the time was a poignant mix of pain and optimism, big band tunes hinted at a big brash future, and anthems to loyal lovers topped the charts. Hard-working Rosie the Riveter battled the languorous "sweater girls" like Lana Turner for not only column inches but also for the hearts and wedding rings of soldiers returning home from war. Betty Grable, the "girl with the million-dollar legs", had her visage and heavily insured gams painted on the nose cones of fighter airplanes—and so the fantasy era of the bombshell was born.

With nylon in scarce supply due to the need for fabric for parachutes, women would paint trompe l'oleil lines up the back of their legs to mimic seamed stockings. Makeup was the ultimate luxury and equalizer: a well-placed swipe of scarlet lipstick and a sweet cloud of perfume could transform a factory worker into a goddess.

As the war ended, prosperity returned, and along with it a jubilant and urgent sense of consumerism. The suburban lifestyle beckoned with all that it entailed. Cars were bigger, sleeker, and faster, spacious ranch style homes replaced cramped apartments, and the cocktail culture reigned supreme. Women went back to ruling the home instead of the factories. They spent their days cooking up elaborate casseroles, being entertained by that new invention television, or frequenting the salon, where their hair was trimmed, teased, and otherwise transformed. Fashion was an impractical combination of cinched waists, petticoats, and kitten heels.

If the 1950s were a crossroads of classic values, counterculture, and cool, the 1960s were an awakening to diverse images of beauty and culture. The hip British influence of Carnaby Street and a little thing called Beatlemania gripped the country. Hemlines rose along with the nation's consciousness. Long hair and bra burning became symbols of female rebellion against centuries of stringent societal beauty tyranny. Makeup was no longer meant to hide a woman's face, but rather to enhance it. (Though somehow light blue eye shadow sneaked into the equation.) Women didn't quite roar just yet, but they were more politcally active than ever before, and working toward the equality in both the home and the workplace. Makeup, fragrance, and other beauty products have long been more than just a fleeting fad. Oscar Wilde opined that beauty was a form of genius, and indeed, using pots of creams, dyes, and powders to transform one's features is nothing short of alchemy—a form of sorcery that women have practiced for thousands of years.

It is a universally acknowledged truth that a woman in pursuit of a man will do nearly anything within her power to make herself more attractive to him. Egyptian women painted their faces with minerals to highlight their best features and anointed their bodies with sweet-smelling oils. In other words, 2,500 or so years before Stonehenge was erected, women were doing their darnedest to stand out from the prehistoric crowd. One might even argue that some cave paintings might have been early billboards chronicling the mating rituals between hunters and gatherers.

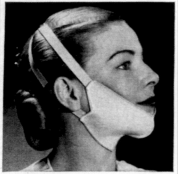

Amazing New Chin and Throat Strap!

15 Minutes a Day Brings Thrilling New Loveliness!

Fast forward several thousand years to the Far East, when rice powder was used to even out features, or ancient Greece where lead powder was used to whiten skin. The practice of using lethal ingredients in beauty treatments ran the gamut from mercury-laden powder used by the Egyptians, to women in sixteenth-century Italy using poisonous belladonna to dilate their pupils, to the arsenic-laced powders of the Elizabethans, to depilatories in the last century which, among other active ingredients, contained rat poison. Painful beauty rituals spanning cultures and centuries range from bound feet to whalebone corsets and girdles. So while it wasn't a brand new concept for women to suffer for beauty, it was in fact a newer concept to advertise it.

The late 1800s saw the launch of women's magazines including *Ladies Home Journal*, *Life*, *Cosmopolitan*, and *Vogue*. In 1891, Nathan Fowler, an editor of *Advertising Age* magazine, recommended that advertising be geared toward women who made most of the buying decisions. And that's when the fun really began. In the early twentieth century, radical fashions and fishnet stockings were imported from France, and Hollywood was declared the official filmmaking mecca and, consequently, the birthplace of fashion icons. The consumption for household toiletries and drugs rose to an estimated $765 million in 1920—the same year that the Nineteenth Amendment was ratified, giving women the right to vote. Women were enjoying previously unheard of freedoms and fashions. They were finding more news that was relevant to them and their lifestyles, more icons to emulate, and more enticements to spend money on their favorite magazines.

By the 1940s and 1950s advertising geared toward women had nearly evolved into an art form. Jim Edwards, a senior editor at *Brandweek* magazine, explains that the beauty ads of that era had a narrative and told a story. Type was as important as imagery in illustrating a product's benefits. Humor, wit, and playfulness didn't enter the equation until the 1960s when the "creative revolution" in advertising took place. Edwards explains, "The older ads were text-heavy, huckster-ish snake-oil pitches. In the modern look today, images dominate and are communicated with a single memorable idea. The new ones are about feelings and emotions."

Advertising and beauty products have to stay on top of the changing sentiments of a given time period. The average woman in the early part of the mid-century was well-groomed, impeccably dressed, and rarely seen in public without her battle armor. Her soft curves were encased in a constricting girdle, and her permed, waved, or lacquered hair was frequently topped with a clever chapeau. Sweater sets were paired with pearls, ladylike gloves were meant to match both the "costume" and the season, and shoes were meticulously coordinated with handbags. Her daily war paint included a layer of foundation, sleekly lined eyes, and a daintily powdered nose, with a girlish pink or perfect red pout to complete the picture. For sweater girls longing for love with their own Deans, Bogeys, and Brandos, looking the part meant *getting* the part—of girlfriend, wife, and mother. Fashion designer Belinda Dickson, who is inspired by the debutantes like Grace Kelly and Jackie Kennedy, admits that in the 1940s and 1950s and in our times as well, "subconsciously, we want to look good for men," be it in our choice of sexy lingerie (like her bespoke cashmere panties) or artfully applied makeup.

Based on the prevalence of bridal imagery in advertising of the times, if you played your cards right your new lipstick could actually get you married! After all, how could he possibly resist your adorably powdered nose courtesy of a "Date Case," or tantalizing ruby lips thanks to "Tape" lipstick by Max Factor, whose tag line was "Sure to tie him up." Cosmetic formulations were New! Exciting! and promised to make you Luminous! Shimmering! and Glamorous! For the first time ads were touched by the glamour of Hollywood. Max Factor used his knowledge of the world of film to promise the ordinary woman she could be transformed into a star.

Cosmetic products, like much of the population, veered between established stereotypes and future-forward formulations and ideals. Lipstick had names like "Futurama" and "Hi-Fi;" face powders included ingredients like silk, silicone, and magic. It was the era of the lavish design; from cars to cosmetic compacts, more was definitely more. Daniela Rinaldi, beauty controller of U.K. luxury goods emporium Harvey Nichols, puts it this way: "In the 1950s and 1960s we decided what the future looks like." Lush, ornate, and sleek, with an eye for fine design and clever detail, we look to the past when we envision the future of cosmetics packaging and design.

Then came the mid 1960s, when women became comfortable letting their hair down—literally and figuratively. The 1960s were a time of unprecedented freedom for women, and their beauty products reflected this. Gone were heavy cosmetic formulations. In their place were sheer formulations, lighter colors, and sleeker packaging made to match their newer lifestyle. For the first time in modern history, women excelled at rebellion. The new aesthetic was young, fresh, and unpredictable. According to Joy Behar, a co-host of *The View*, "The sixties were aberrational in that young women gave in and learned to love their natural attributes."

So where does that leave us today? While advertising imagery and messages may have evolved, the emotions evinced are the same: these products will make you more beautiful, attractive, and alluring. So should women try to resist the messages? Not according to cosmetics entrepreneur Bobbi Brown. "Beauty advertising is inspirational, and every woman wants to be pretty." Advertising trends come and go, and much has changed since the days of the

You create new glamour with Beauty Tone Bulbs!

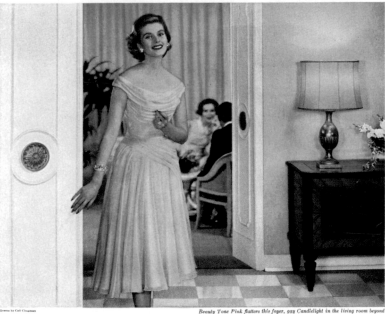

Gowns by Ceil Chapman

Beauty Tone Pink flatters this foyer, gay Candlelight in the living room beyond

Here's *new magic for your home*—brought to you first by Westinghouse. A complete range of tinted bulbs —to make colors *wake up and sing!* Exclusive sealed-in tints, soft and subtle. Lovely to live with . . . easy to see by. You'll create new glamour for *pennies* with this Westinghouse Beauty Tone™ trio. *Buy all three . . . for flattery!*

YOU CAN BE SURE...IF IT'S

Westinghouse

Westinghouse Beauty Tone Pink . . . new flattery for every complexion, for unsuspected loveliness in fabrics and wallpapers! But buy all *three* Beauty Tone tints—they do wonderful things for your home and you.

Westinghouse Beauty Tone Aqua . . . "opens up" small areas, subdues confining colors. This refreshing, subtle tint was *decorator selected*, is "decorator-right!" Restfully glare-free to read by too!

Westinghouse Beauty Tone Candlelight . . . so welcoming and gay! Brings out richness of woodwork, accents warm colors in fabrics . . . creates a festive party atmosphere that makes it even more fun to entertain.

"This Season . . . Change your lighting for more glamourous living."
Buy long-lasting Beauty Tone bulbs in 60, 75, 100, 150 watts and 3-way sizes.

mid-century beauty icons, in Brown's opinion. "It is not about cookie cutter beauty anymore. There are a lot more options now." Options that include evolving body types, international features, and less specific ideals of beauty.

Rita Gam was a 1952 Golden Globe nominee, a *Life* magazine cover girl, and bridesmaid for Grace Kelly. In her current incarnation she serves as the executive producer and host of a PBS series called *World Beauty*, which explores the concept of beauty around the world. She admits that for her, the makeup and trappings of celebrity were part of a role that she played—the role of starlet. Real beauty, she believes, has nothing to do with physical beauty. Rather, she says, "Beauty is what you do and what you accomplish." In real life, "beauty is an ingredient in fashion for the contemporary woman. It's how you present yourself to the world in the era that you're in."

Beauty advertising of the 1940s–1960s era favored models with porcelain skin tones. Dorothy Dandridge, Rita Moreno, Sophia Loren, and Rita Hayworth might have symbolized a mélange of cultures and complexions, but it was invariably the Grace Kelly, Sandra Dee, or Natalie Wood ideal that was used to pitch products. While the three famously feuding grande dames of the cosmetic industry, Estée Lauder, Elizabeth Arden, and Helena Rubenstein were short, dark, and aggressive, the advertising norm for that generation were sleek, mostly blonde Breck girls or lily white Ivory Soap girls.

In our own multi-cultural society, beauty ideals have evolved to a certain degree. Claudine Ingeri, bookings editor for *Elle* magazine, chooses all of the models used in the magazine's fashion shoots. She explains that while traditional beauty, including "almond shaped eyes, high cheekbones, a great body, and a great smile," will always remain the ideal, our concept of the ideal has also evolved since the mid-century when bland beauty was an accepted archetype. In our own times personality and energy are just as essential. Ingeri meets hundreds of models but acknowledges that their defining qualities have to be energy and personality, because "people get really beautiful really fast, or really ugly really fast depending on their energy."

So has that much changed in the generations from Marilyn to Madonna? Yes and no. We still believe in the concept of hope in a jar. We still seek salvation from shadows and rescue from wrinkles. New ad campaigns may boast "real" women instead of models, but we know that it's a matter of time until the unrealistic ideal returns to the pages of our favorite glossy magazines. At worst, the beauty industry can encourage a cult of insecurity with women becoming obsessed with the hopes of looking more beautiful. At best, the search for the newest formulations, colors, and textures can inspire women to create their own unique brand of beauty, even if the billboard kind is unattainable. Bob Froese, president of the Denver-based advertising agency The Brainstorm Group, sums it up this way, "Even when women know that they'll never actually achieve that kind of beauty, there's something comforting in being gorgeous by association!"

Well, hello gorgeous!

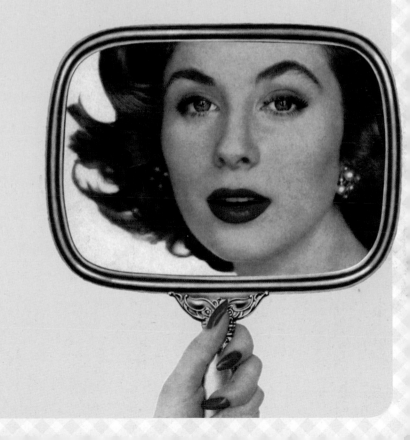

Chapter One
A Youthful Complexion

✦✦✦◆▣◆✦✦✦

Ask any beauty insider the real secret to allure and they'll likely wax rhapsodic about luminous, healthy skin. Cosmetic industry consultant Kim-Van Dang, president of KVDNYC, who spent six years as beauty director of *In Style* magazine, advises that it isn't about covering up, it's about enhancing what you already have—especially great skin. After all, "if you have great skin, you need very little makeup." And for generations, women have feverishly pursued the holy grail of flawless skin.

Since ancient times, women have fantasized about the proverbial fountain of youth, though in recent years the quest for younger-looking skin has become something of a national obsession. In generations past, skin care treatments were mainly perfumed softeners; as science progressed, so did ingredients, formulations, and price tags. A recent report states the international cosmetics industry is worth about $150 billion annually, with the most money being spent on skincare and anti-aging treatments. To put this in historical perspective, in 1949, the annual income hovered at considerably below $2,000 per capita. In our own times, there are face creams and treatments that retail for $2,500 for a monthly supply. Women are spending more money than ever before to keep their complexions looking young and supple.

Skin care products of the 1940s, 1950s, and 1960s had heavy formulations, perfumes, tints, and colors that weren't frequently found in nature. Pancake makeup all but obscured the skin's natural allure, and removing makeup involved goopy cold creams or drying soaps. These products glowingly gushed to provide "skin like a teenager," "movie star skin," or better skin in a matter of days—guaranteed!

Before Coco Chanel first popularized the deep tan, perfectly pale skin was the ideal, with exaggerated eye makeup, doll-like blush, and muted lips. Swinging Carnaby Street girls were famed for the pale porcelain complexion so revered in London and beyond. Bronzed flesh was the aesthetic domain of construction workers and the so-called lower class.

Elizabeth Hughes, formerly a Tokyo-based reporter for the *San Francisco Examiner*, observes that Japanese women are still most passionate about their skin and routinely use skin-whitening products. She describes their preoccupation with sun protection: "Protective gear goes beyond parasols, hats, and gloves to UV-blocking protective fabric fashioned into sleeves and stoles."

Then came the 1960s, when the California beach culture reigned, and the expression "healthy tan" wasn't a contradiction in terms but rather the desired norm. Women all over the states yearned to have the healthy coloring of Annette Funicello or Gidget and did everything possible to try to morph into the mythical "California Girl" so worshiped by the Beach Boys. Advertisements gleefully encouraged women to "Tan Gloriously with Skol!" and to "Get that glorious summer-tan look… GE Sunlamp tans like the sun!" with nary a mention of long-term damage, wrinkling, or any of those icky aging side effects.

In the 1960s, women would liberally baste themselves in baby oil and position light reflectors on their faces, thus ensuring that they soaked up a maximum amount of UV rays. In our own times, the daughters and granddaughters of these sun-damaged baby boomers find themselves addicted to anti-aging skin care serums, lotions, and treatments. Today skin tinting is competing with tanning salons for the best way to fake the sun. Skin tinting trends run the gamut from gilded peach to St. Tropez bronze, and sophisticated self-tanning products range from gels to lotions to airbrushing.

According to anti-aging specialist Dr. Nicholas Perricone, there really hasn't been much change in the skincare industry up until about five years ago. With the advent of "cosmeceuticals," or skin care treatments containing active, pharmaceutical-grade components, women could do more than offer their ravaged skin a temporary fix—they could work toward healing it. Perricone advocates a three-pronged approach to great skin care: a balanced diet, supplements, and skincare products to suit your skin type. Perricone cites the restorative benefits of fresh fruit and vegetables, and enough sleep and exercise to keep you looking radiant.

While many women are turning to high-tech skin care solutions, some are sticking to tried and true folk remedies to keep their glowing complexions. For years it has been rumored that her royal highness Queen Elizabeth II drinks a daily infusion of barley water to keep her natural glow. And indeed, her skin appears to be as flawless now as when she was a young woman in the 1950s. David Pogson, a senior press officer at Buckingham Palace would neither confirm nor deny this speculation. Instead he said, "There is so much known about the Queen that we have to respect the parts that she wishes to maintain for herself—her beauty and hair regime."

How refreshing to know that in a world of reality television, instant-blogging, and immediate media, for some public figures, beauty and skin-care secrets will always remain sacred.

New Palmolive Soap Gives New Life to Your Complexion!

JUST ONE BAR WILL PROVE IT! BECAUSE NEW PALMOLIVE
BRINGS OUT BEAUTY WHILE IT CLEANS YOUR SKIN!

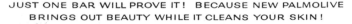

New Lather!

**Think of the
softest, creamiest lather!**
It's yours in New Palmolive.
Rich, white lather that actually soothes
as it cleanses... helps your *true*
complexion beauty come through!

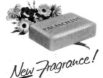

New Fragrance!

**Think of the most
fabulous French perfumes!**
They were the inspiration
for Palmolive's haunting new
fragrance. So fresh, so clean,
so heaven-scented!

New Color!

**Think of the
fresh green of spring!**
That's the color of
New Palmolive...all
pretty and new
for a prettier you!

New Wrapper!

**Wrap them all up
in gleaming emerald foil**
—and there you have
the exciting New Palmolive Soap
...the best news your
complexion ever had!

There's never been a beauty soap like this before... **NOT EVEN PALMOLIVE!**

Wonderful Dial Soap!

For the woman who's afraid to use

soap on her face, Dial is a revelation. For while
Dial removes the bacteria that often spread
skin blemishes, Dial is mild. Wonderful Dial!

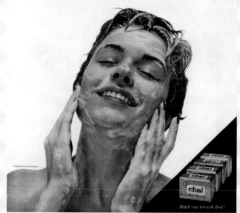

Match your tile with Dial!

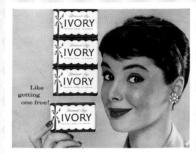

Like getting one free!

4 for the price of 3

*P*rocter & Gamble's White
Soap got a new name, Ivory
Soap, when company founder
Harley Procter was inspired by the
45th Psalm, which stated: "All thy
garments smell of myrrh, and aloes,
and cassia, out of ivory palaces,
whereby they have made thee glad."

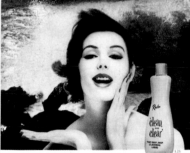

Look!..a startlingly different facial cleanser
—*foams* dirt out...*foams* moisture in!

You'll *see* the difference!... *feel* the difference!... *look* the difference!

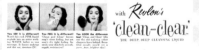

with *Revlon's*

'clean and clear'

THE DEEP, DEEP CLEANSING LIQUID

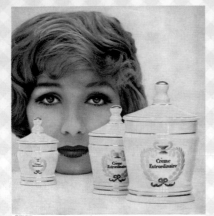

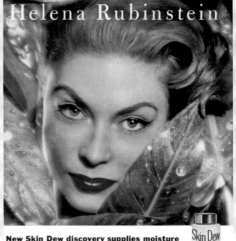

Lux
I love
you

Your moisturizing creamy lather lets me wash without dry skin worries!

One of Nars Cosmetics top-selling products is a peachy tinted blush called Orgasm. One imagines that it is meant to mimic the flushed skin and satisfied glow exhibited during, um, orgasm.

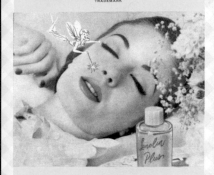
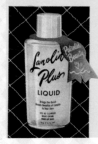

19

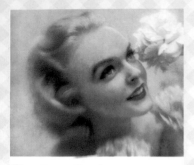

That Ivory Look—so clear...so fresh ...so easily yours

A complexion smooth and clear—petal-soft and fresh! That's what the magic of Ivory's mildness can give to you. Just make a simple change to regular care with this soap that's mild enough for a baby's skin, and meet your complexion will improve. You'll like the new freshness—the *new* texture—the smoother feel. You'll like *That Ivory Look!*

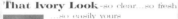

More doctors advise Ivory than any other soap

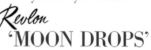

*M*ax Factor touted his makeup as having near magical qualities. Skin was said to look so flawless that it was nearly impossible to tell where makeup began or ended.

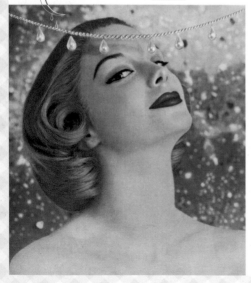

YOU DON'T <u>TELL</u> YOUR AGE...WHY SHOW IT?

Take 2 minutes a day to take years off your looks!

Revlon 'MOON DROPS'

...1 minute in the morning to smooth on 'Moon Drops' as a makeup foundation for a dewy skin all day.

...1 minute at night to give your skin a deep "drink" of 'Moon Drops' (greaseless, quickly absorbed.)

Start tonight!...Give back to your skin the natural oils and moisture of youth

After 25, your skin loses youth's moisture day by day. Greasy creams give little help—they can't penetrate as 'Moon Drops' can. For here at last is a liquid that moisturizes as it lubricates. Its secret: a new balance of humectants; plus Lanolite. Both . . . *only in 'Moon Drops'!*

Works both OUTSIDE and INSIDE the skin to bring a *profound* turnabout in your looks.

OUTSIDE: 'Moon Drops' thin molecular film *attracts moisture from the air*, holds it in your skin! Protects against drying effects of sun, wind.

INSIDE: This same invisible film preserves healthy moisture *inside the skin from "aging" evaporation.*

So little does so much—so quickly! Yes, use only a few drops each time. Your reward: dewy-freshness, a smoother, younger-looking skin.

3.00 and 5.00 (plus tax)

'MOON DROPS'—THE MAGICAL MOISTURIZER FOR DRY OR AGING SKIN

20

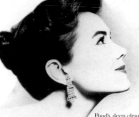

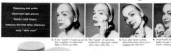

In recent years Alpha Hydroxy Acids (AHAs), which include lactic acids, have been added to costly skin treatments used to treat wrinkles. One of Cleopatra's famous beauty secrets was bathing in spoiled milk—from which lactic acids are derived.

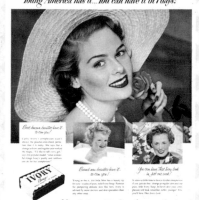

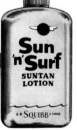

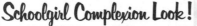

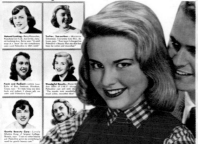

Here's a recipe for a barley water infusion from www.goodybaggifts.com that is reported to give your skin a natural glow: Soak 1/2 cup of barley in hot water. Discard barley. Add 1 teaspoon honey and the juice of a lemon to the water and drink.

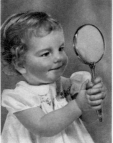

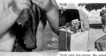

How Judy, *age 1*
taught Jane, *age 22*
to look <u>more</u> beautiful

"JUDY JANE WAS CRYING. She jerked my carriage sorta mad like and mumured, 'It isn't fair. You with that perfect complexion... when *I'm* the one who needs it... to get a few beaus!' I did so want to help her. But—I was speechless!"

"'I WAS SO EMBARRASSED when Dr. Gordon called. He winked at her and said to me, 'Hello beautiful! That Ivory Soap I advised certainly helps keep you lovely!' Sensitive skin doctor busy—'I want to—but skin just perked up—"

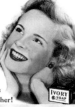

"'SHE THOUGHT I WAS ASLEEP that night when she sneaked in to borrow my Ivory. I wanted to tell her mom doctors advise Ivory Soap than all other brands together. And that Ivory has no coloring, confusion, so strong perhaps that might be irritating. But... words failed me!"

"'SHE THOUGHT I WAS ASLEEP again 2 weeks later when she came in with her new boy friend and whispered, 'Thanks for the tip about Ivory, Judy. Since I've changed to gentle Ivory cleansing, my complexion's ever so much lovelier!'"
90¾in"), pure —N. Harris.

Look lovelier... with pure, mild
IVORY...the soap more Doctors
advise than all other brands together!

IVORY SOAP

It's the new double-action cleanser that cleans and moisturizes
to the depths of your skin. It smooths away the
day's gathering of make-up, oil and dirt as it moisturizes
deep-down...leaving your face flawlessly clean
and fresh, never dry or dull. Just $1, ...TREAT YOURSELF TO BEAUTY...TUSSY

Liquid Pearl
treasures your complexion

©1956 Tussy, 485 Park Avenue, New York

Liquid Pearl
NEW DOUBLE-ACTION
FOR ALL SKIN TYPES
TUSSY

Now! Exclusive screening formula
gives you

a Lovelier Tan

Swimsuit by Catalina

Only Skol brings you this marvelous new
tanning formula—lets you tan faster,
more beautifully than ever!

● Skol's two exclusive screening ingredients *let you control* your tanning scientifically! When you cover yourself with
Skol you draw a protective curtain between you and the "danger rays" of the
sun. You don't blister. You don't get a
disfiguring red-burn.

Yet Skol's new formula allows pre-
cisely enough of the sun's "tanning rays"
through to give you a *lovely, flattering
tan*—the most glorious tan of your life.
Get non-oily Skol—also available in
plastic bottles.

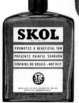

SKOL
PROMOTES A BENEFICIAL TAN
PREVENTS PAINFUL SUNBURN
CONTAINS NO GREASE—NOT OILY

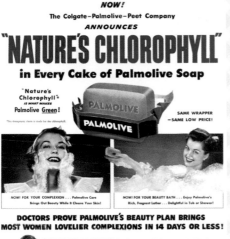
Unusual zit zappers include, dabbing white toothpaste on spots, washing skin with dishwashing liquid, dotting with eye drops to remove redness, and covering with honey and a bandage overnight.

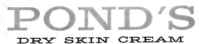

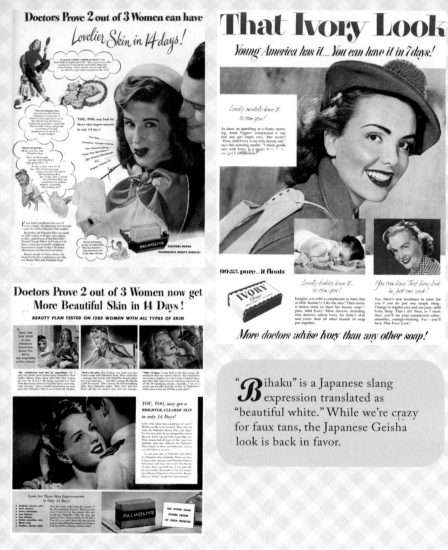

Doctors Prove 2 out of 3 Women can have
Lovelier Skin in 14 days!

That Ivory Look
Young America has it... You can have it in 7 days!

Doctors Prove 2 out of 3 Women now get More Beautiful Skin in 14 Days !

"*B*ihaku" is a Japanese slang expression translated as "beautiful white." While we're crazy for faux tans, the Japanese Geisha look is back in favor.

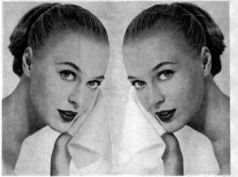

Scotties facial tissues—so soft to your skin, yet so *strong*

What makes **Scotties** so wonderful for removing make-up? ...**Wet-strength!**

Soft as Scotties are, Scotties hold together —even when you're using liquid cleansers. Prove it with this dramatic "jewel" test ▸

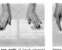

Pour two pools of liquid cleansing cream. Soak a tissue without the wet-strength of Scotties in one pool, a Scottie in the other.

Tissue without wet-strength breaks! Cream-soaked tissue without the wet-strength of Scotties breaks when you drop just one earring into it.

Scottie doesn't break! Drop two earrings, bracelet, pin, necklace and cream-soaked Scottie—and it doesn't break! Scotties have wet-strength.

Take off make-up the glamorous new way—with Scotties in powderpuff pink, white, yellow

SCOTTIES FACIAL TISSUES—ANOTHER FINE PAPER PRODUCT BY SCOTT

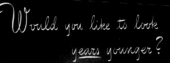

Would you like to look years younger?

OILS of the WILDERNESS

Don't count your age by birthdays . . . a woman is as young as she looks. See how, in just 20 to 30 minutes, Oils of the Wilderness helps bring younger looking beauty. See how wonderfully this lipoid cream aids skin shadowed by lines, marred by roughness or lack of firm contours; often the tattletale signs of lipoid deficiency. Pat the cream over your face and throat. Watch how quickly your skin can absorb the wonder-working lipoids. It's a streamlined beauty treatment indeed. $5. *plus tax*

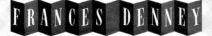

FRANCES DENNEY

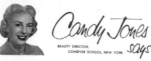

Candy Jones *says*

BEAUTY DIRECTOR,
CONOVER SCHOOL, NEW YORK

"Watch your skin thrive on Cashmere Bouquet Soap!"

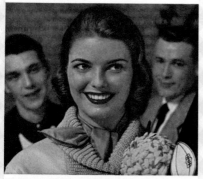

Who's winning all the attention? "It can be *you* . . . if you give your skin 3-way beauty care with Cashmere Bouquet Soap," says Candy Jones.

Cleans cleaner than creams. Your skin is so much cleaner when you use Cashmere Bouquet! No cream film!

Stimulates with no astringent sting, as you stroke Cashmere Bouquet's mild lather over your skin.

Softens without lotion stickiness. Leaves normal, dry or oily skin naturally softer, smoother! No sticky feel!

Give your skin this 3-way beauty care!

No more bother with greasy cleansing creams, sticky lotions and stinging astringents! *Now*, with just a cake of Cashmere Bouquet Soap, you can give your skin the beauty care of famous Conover students. This wonderful 3-way beauty care actually *cleans cleaner than creams* . . . *stimulates gently* . . . *softens and smooths your skin, too*. Just like using a whole row of beauty products . . . but so much quicker and easier. Start today, and watch your skin thrive!

Cashmere Bouquet
TOILET SOAP

REGULAR
OR BIG BATH SIZE

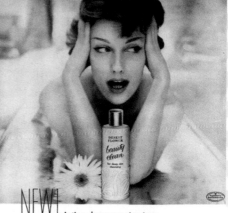

NEW! Lotion-cleanser <u>moisturizes</u> as it flows out <u>hidden</u> dirt!

Now! Your skin can be *pure* in every pore—cleaner, softer, smoother than ever before! Almost any cleanser—soap, cream or liquid—will clean the visible top layer of your skin. But new, deep-down BEAUTY CLEAN can clean the unseen! Here's a new kind of clean: a lavish lotion that works with the speed of light—takes a deep plunge to penetrate far, far below your skin's surface—flows out hidden dirt and makeup—leaves your skin tingling-clean, misted with delicious, young moisture—with a new, precious, poreless look! No drying, trying soaps or detergents in BEAUTY CLEAN, instead, it lavishes your face to petal-soft, fine-textured freshness. Begin tonight to be more beautiful tomorrow!

$1^{25}_{plus tax}$

DESERT FLOWER

beauty clean

by **SHULTON**

*W*omen of the war era took tea baths to fake a golden tan, realizing perhaps that the tannins in darker tealeaves could temporarily stain skin.

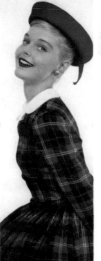
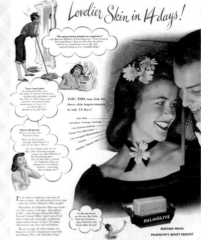
> *H*elena Rubenstein was said to have advised the use of layers of freshly sliced meat as a refreshing facial mask.

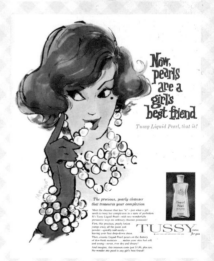

Even before 25

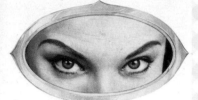

dry-skin lines begin to show

Sometimes as early as 19—a woman's skin can start to dry out—look older! You see it around your eyes—tiny crow's feet, feathery crinkles, crepe-y dryness.

To prevent the "middle-aging" effects of dry skin—*you must replace natural skin oils every day!*

Exceptionally rich in homogenized lanolin, Pond's Dry Skin Cream instantly restores softening oils to parched skin . . . smooths out tiny dry lines. And its special moisturizing action softens away flaky dryness . . . keeps your skin looking dewy-soft and young!

Soften away dry crow's feet—gently tap Pond's Dry Skin Cream under eyes and at outside corners. This special cream is *extra rich in lanolin* . . . freshens "tired" dry skin, smooths dry crinkles quickly

Smooth parched, crepe-y skin—lightly pat this satiny cream over the eyelids. The rich lanolin in Pond's Dry Skin Cream is *homogenized* to penetrate faster, deeper. Dry skin literally *drinks in* its richness

Ease out dry "frown lines"—smooth Pond's Dry Skin Cream up between eyes, out over brows. Unlike a thin, runny liquid that just "surface-oils" dry skin, this rich-textured cream softens deeply. Use generously—a season's supply is less than a dollar!

Extra Rich in
HOMOGENIZED LANOLIN
for faster, deeper softening

So effective— more women use it than any other dry skin care

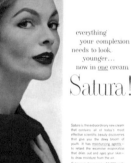

everything your complexion needs to look younger . . . now in *one* cream

Satura!

Satura is the extraordinary new cream that contains all of today's most effective scientific beauty discoveries that give you the dewy bloom of youth. It has *moisturizing agents*—to retard the excessive evaporation that dries out and ages your skin—to draw moisture from the air.

Estrogenic hormones—10,000 units in each ounce—actively work beneath the skin . . . to help smooth and cushion away tiny wrinkles.

And Satura has *Vitamin A* . . . which staunchly guards against dry flakiness.

Tonight and every night . . . smooth on a film of silky pink Satura. It disappears . . . starts working instantly.

Satura magnet: smooth on a time of Satura every morning, under make-up.

For beauty the modern way .... Dorothy Gray

30

SUNBURN

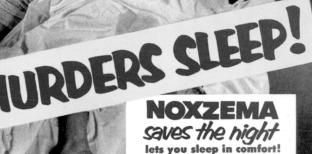

MURDERS SLEEP!

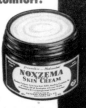

Doctors Prove 2 out of 3 Women can have More Beautiful Skin in 14 Days!

14-Day Palmolive Plan tested on 1285 women with all types of skin!

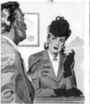

READ THIS TRUE STORY of what the Proved 14-Day Palmolive Plan did for Harriett Edwards of Chicago, Illinois

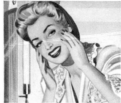

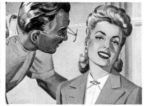

"My complexion had lost its soft, smooth look. So I said 'yes' when I was invited to try the new 14-Day Palmolive Plan—along with 1284 other women all over the U.S.A.! My group reported to a Chicago skin doctor. Some of us had dry skins; some oily; some 'average.' After a careful examination, we were given the Palmolive Plan to use *at home* for 14 days.

"Here's the proved Palmolive Plan: Wash your face 3 times a day with Palmolive Soap. Then—each time —massage your clean face with that lovely, soft Palmolive beauty-lather . . . just like a cream. Do this for a *full* 60 seconds. This massage extracts the full beautifying effect from Palmolive lather for your skin. Then rinse and dry. That's all!

"After 14 days, I went back to my doctor. He confirmed what my mirror told me. My skin was smoother, finer, less oily! Later I learned *many* skin improvements had been observed by all the 36 examining doctors. Actually 2 out of 3 of all the 1285 women got see-able, feel-able results. So the 14-Day Palmolive Plan is now my beauty plan for life!"

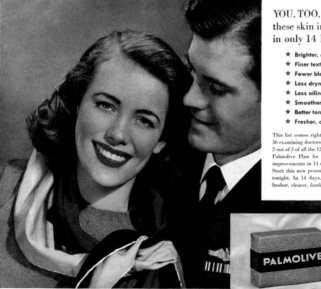

YOU, TOO, may look for these skin improvements in only 14 Days!

★ Brighter, cleaner skin
★ Finer texture
★ Fewer blemishes
★ Less dryness
★ Less oiliness
★ Smoother skin
★ Better tone
★ Fresher, clearer color

This list comes right from the reports of the 36 examining doctors! Their records show that 2 out of 3 of all the 1285 women who tested the Palmolive Plan for you got many of these improvements in 14 days! Now it's *your* turn! Start this new *proved* way of using Palmolive tonight. In 14 days, you, too, may look for fresher, clearer, *lovelier* skin!

PALMOLIVE

NO OTHER SOAP OFFERS PROOF OF SUCH RESULTS!

DON'T WASTE SOAP! Soap uses vital materials needed to win the war!

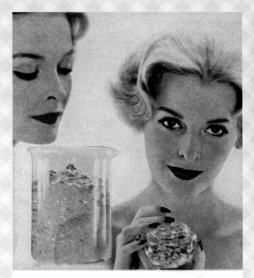

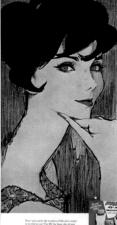

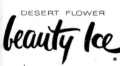
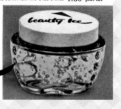
*T*hough she had played the original Eliza Dolittle in the Broadway musical *My Fair Lady*, Julie Andrews wasn't considered pretty enough for the film version, and the coveted part went to Audrey Hepburn.

"Sun-glare" crinkles?

Flaky patches?

Coarsened texture?

Summer's dry skin problems

really show up **now**!

How to **deep-soften** parched, dried-out skin with extra-rich Pond's Dry Skin Cream

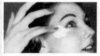

Smooth out "sun-glare" crinkles—Lightly pat Pond's Dry Skin Cream around your eyes. Its extra lanolin-richness is *homogenized* . . . penetrates faster, deeper! Baked-in crow's feet quickly smooth away!

Cream away parched, flaky patches—Firmly circle on this rich cream. Not thin or watery, Pond's Dry Skin Cream has a richness you can actually *feel*. Its lanolin goes *deep*—instantly softens flaky roughness.

Soften coarsened, crepe-y throat—Stroke Pond's Dry Skin Cream up throat. This Cream's *special emulsifier* restores vital moisture to sun-dried, papery skin. Overnight, your skin looks younger, firmer. Get the large jar—*less* than one dollar!

Extra Rich in

HOMOGENIZED LANOLIN

for faster, **deeper** softening

So effective—more women use it than any other dry skin care

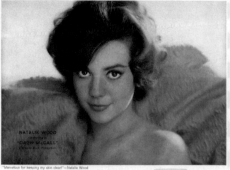

*N*IVEA produced the famous NIVEA TIN with spelling as "Crème" in 1959. NIVEA was so well known that no explanation of what the crème actually did was needed or used on the packaging.

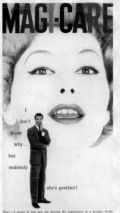

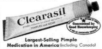
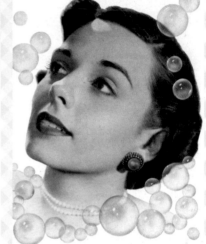
35

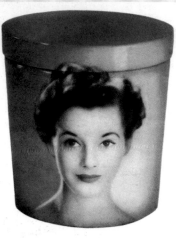

Trust DOROTHY GRAY
for beauty out of the blue...

Dreams are realized, hopes of beauty fulfilled, out of
the blue jars and bottles that bear the Dorothy Gray label.
Because the creams and lotions they contain are *personalized*, for
individual skin types, they reward you far in excess
of the few delightful minutes you devote to their daily use.

FOR NORMAL SKIN—use Salon Cold Cream $1.25 to $4;
Orange Flower Skin Lotion $1 to $3.75;
Special Dry-Skin Mixture $2.25 and $4.

FOR DRY SKIN—use Dry-Skin Cleanser $1.25 to $4;
Orange Flower Skin Lotion $1 to $3.75; and
Special Dry-Skin Mixture $2.25 and $4.

FOR OILY SKIN—use Liquefying Cleansing Cream $1 to $4;
Texture Lotion $1 to $3.75; and Suppling Cream $1 and $2.

FOR COMBINATION (*part dry, part oily*) SKIN—use
Salon Cold Cream $1.25 to $4; Texture Lotion $1 to $3.75;
and Special Dry-Skin Mixture $2.25 and $4.

All prices plus tax.

Trust DOROTHY GRAY...
America's loveliest women do!

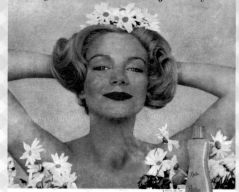

*O*h baby! Use chilled teething rings (one for each eye) to eliminate puffiness around eyes. Use diaper cream on irritated skin and broken capillaries after a night of overindulgence.

Soap operas were originally radio dramas sponsored by soap companies, most notably Procter & Gamble. In 1949, soap operas as we know them were introduced to television.

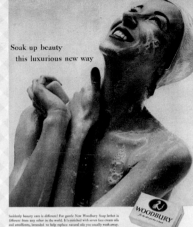

Soak up beauty
this luxurious new way

Suddenly beauty care is different! For gentle New Woodbury Soap lather is different from any other in the world. It's enriched with seven face cream oils and emollients, intended to help replace natural oils you usually wash away. It's wonderful for your complexion. (A blessing for dry skin.) And your bath are sheer luxury — new beauty baths from head to toe. You'll like its delicate floral fragrances. Do try New Woodbury Soap... *for the skin you love to touch!*

WOODBURY

New Woodbury Soap is enriched with 7 face cream oils

That Ivory Look
Young America has it... You can have it in 7 days!

**Well-known beauties have it—
so can you!**

Even in brightest sunlight, cover-girl Jean Moorhead's smooth complexion welcomes close-ups. "But goodness," says Jean, "any girl can keep her complexion clear and sparkling with the help of pure, mild Ivory!" Leading models know—and so should you—there's no substitute for purity and mildness in your complexion soap.

**Brand-new beauties have it—
so can you!**

There's beauty news for you in baby Lorada's flaw-less complexion! It's this: The soap that's safe enough for her skin . . . pure, mild Ivory . . . is right for your complexion. Why, more doctors, including skin doctors, advise Ivory for baby's skin and yours, than all other brands put together!

**You can have That Ivory Look
in just one week!**

Yes, your mirror can reflect a lovelier you that quickly! Here's all you do—just change to regular care and use pure, mild Ivory Soap. Then, in one short week, your complexion will be softer, smoother, actually younger looking! You'll have *That Ivory Look!*

99 44/100% pure...it floats

*More doctors
advise Ivory than
any other soap*

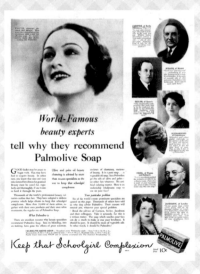

*World-Famous
beauty experts*

tell why they recommend
Palmolive Soap

GOOD looks may be yours to begin with. You may have had to acquire beauty. In either case, you know that one can't just take casual beauty care for granted. Beauty must be cared for, regularly and thoroughly, if you want to hold it through the years.

Thousands of the world's professional beauty experts realize that fact. They have adopted a definite practice which helps obtain to keep that schoolgirl complexion. More than 10,000 of them advise, together with their own products and their own wise treatments, the regular use of Palmolive Soap.

What Palmolive is

There are excellent reasons why beauty specialists recommend Palmolive Soap. Into its blending, into its making, there goes the efforts of great scientists

Olive and palm oil beauty cleansing is advised by most that in care specialists as the way to keep that schoolgirl complexion

motions of chemistry, medicine of beauty. It is a pure soap . . . a vegetable oil soap. Into Palmolive go the oils of olive and palm—no other fats whatever. No artificial coloring matter. Here is an undeniably wholesome soap so one on pure face!

For particular profiles

Six of the world's most prominent specialists are quoted on this page. Thousands of others have told us why they advise Palmolive. Their counsel will reassure you, whatever your special problem.

Read the advice of Carton, Stiller, Jacobson and their colleagues. Take it seriously, for this is a serious matter. Mild soap that can do as much to make as true your loveliness. It should be pure. It should be made of vegetable oils. In other words, it should be Palmolive!

Keep that Schoolgirl Complexion

PALMOLIVE

10¢

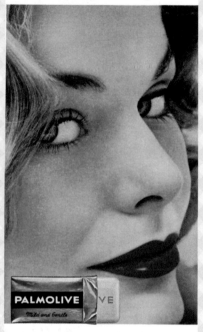

*D*isappointed by a fishing prize won early in her career at Stanley Home Products, Mary Kay Ash went on to create woman-friendly rewards at her own company—including the famous pink Cadillac.

Shhh! your skin is showing *your age!*

You need *Jacqueline Cochran's*

FLOWING VELVET

This modern flowing formula has helped countless women — just like you — who had despaired of a dry, prematurely aging skin.

Jacqueline Cochran has found a whole new answer to the dry-skin problem and its main cause, dehydration of the sub-surface tissues. After years of research, she discovered Hydrolin, a new ingredient that transfers beneficial moisture into the deep tissues of the skin. Thanks to exclusive Hydrolin...and other rich components, Jacqueline Cochran created an entirely new kind of 3-way beauty formula.

Unique Flowing Velvet acts 3-ways:

- *It furnishes moisture that actually sinks into your skin.*
- *It provides necessary oils for essential lubrication.*
- *It maintains the normal balance of oils and moisture.*

One touch mirrors the beautiful change! Tiny lines smooth out, years seem to melt away! Use Flowing Velvet day and night. It is hormone-free, *greaseless,* won't smear your make-up or smudge your pillow.

See for yourself. Make Flowing Velvet your 24-hour beauty care... and see how much younger and lovelier you can look. Why not start today!

The one-and-only
Jacqueline Cochran's
FLOWING VELVET
**the tested and proven moisture-giving formula
for maturing, sensitive and drying skins**

At fine stores everywhere.

3⁰⁰
5⁰⁰
8⁵⁰ *and*
15⁰⁰
plus tax

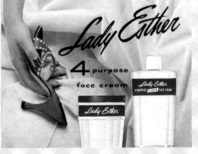

AT LAST! YOU CAN

Stop "Make-Up Damage"

to your skin!

● Ordinary skin cleansers were never made for modern make-ups!

New-formula Lady Esther 4-Purpose Face Cream is the modern cream especially blended to clean, soften, refine, and protect your complexion from the clogging, drying, aging effects of make-up!

Try it tonight — cream or liquid. Then sleep tight, with a radiantly clean skin safe from "make-up damage."

Lady Esther

4 purpose
face cream

39

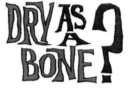

DRY AS A BONE?

Wish for **Tussy** *Dry Skin Cream*

Flakes and flurries give you worries?
Don't try to wash away dryness troubles
with teardrops . . . cleanse your delicate
skin with Tussy Dry Skin Cream!
It's made just for a princess like you who feels
that too much summer sun and wind have
touched her cheek. This gentle cleanser coaxes
make-up and dirt away quick as a wish. Then the
special blend of moisturizers and lubricants
goes right to work chasing dryness from sight!
Promise your complexion you'll cleanse with
Dry Skin Cream happily ever after . . . just $1.25,
plus tax, for a big jar of wishes-come-true.

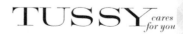

TUSSY *cares for you*

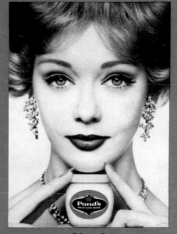

YOU'RE NEVER TOO YOUNG TO

Start building Beauty

Once you built with blocks. But you're a big girl now . . . you play with beauty and build it on your youth. Many a deb dream-skin has had its beginnings in Velva Cream. Many a grown girl is grateful for her date-full of Ardena Junior Essentials. Better begin now to cleanse . . . refresh . . . smooth, night and morning. To make-up, too, with Elizabeth Arden. To realize that the best beauty preparations are an economy in the end.

ARDENA CLEANSING CREAM, 1.00 to 6.00 • ARDENA SKIN LOTION, 85c to 12.00 • ARDENA VELVA CREAM, 1.50 to 6.00
FEATHERLIGHT FOUNDATION, 1.50 • CREAM ROUGE, 1.25, 1.75 • LIGHT ILLUSION POWDER, 1.75, 3.00 • LIP PENCIL, 1.00, 1.50, 2.00 • NAIL LACQUER, 1.00
All prices plus taxes

Elizabeth Arden

N oxzema launched Cover Girl Cosmetics in 1960 as medicated makeup for teens and younger women.

beautiful discovery!

New!
Moisture Base
by Pond's

new kind of <u>greaseless</u> foundation cream!
brings you "night cream" moisturizing
under your make-up all day!

Creates an all-day "moisture reserve." At last a cream that goes beyond superficial smoothing . . . that actually controls the moisture level of your skin *under* your make-up. At the same time, it normalizes your skin's protective chemistry all day long.

Prevents under-make-up dryout! New Pond's Moisture Base protects your skin against sun and wind—the drying effects of make-up itself! Your skin stays soft and dewy all day.

For a smooth, no-shine finish. Pond's Moisture Base is greaseless. Your skin never feels sticky—your make-up never streaks or cakes. Completely transparent, it can't conflict with any make-up shade.

For a lovelier face, smooth on New Pond's Moisture Base every morning. And, of course, use it for nighttime moisturizing, too.

Pond's Moisture Base
NEW GREASELESS UNDER-MAKE-UP MOISTURIZER

41

A NEW "INVISIBLE" CREAM THAT COMPLETELY PREVENTS SUNBURN

as no suntan oil or lotion can!

Contains science's most powerful sun screen . . .
shuts out all the sun's burning rays . . .
specially developed by dermatologists

Now . . . Stop painful, ugly "spot burning"!

No need to look like a lady from Mars

Protect nose, lips, shoulders, other "tender skin" areas—without using disfiguring nose shades, white ointments!

If your nose turns poppy red again and again—if your lips tend to blister painfully, or nose, shoulders and backs of knees red-burn *even through a tan*, Skolex is for you. A thin "invisible" film on "tender skin" areas lets you stay in the sun for hours—without experiencing the slightest burning or reddening!

Now . . . Spend all day in the sun!

No danger of glare burn

Go golfing, fishing, or on boating trips without fear of overexposure!

Even though your skin is winter-white—you can face your first sail, your first fishing trip of the season, without any fear of burning or blistering. Skolex contains the most powerful sun screen known to science—keeps your skin *out of the sun*, completely protected from the direct burning rays or the reflected glare of sun on water. Skolex is greaseless, odorless, "disappears" from your skin without leaving a visible trace.

Now . . . Heliophobes—go out in the sun!

For those whose skin can't take the sun, absolute protection against painful burning, rashes, blisters, due to sun allergies.

Skolex has brought new freedom to people who are allergic to the sun. Now for the first time, millions of sun allergy sufferers can enjoy outdoor fun, without fear of the misery that would ordinarily follow such exposure. Hundreds of leading dermatologists throughout the country have recommended Skolex to their patients.

New freedom for sun allergy sufferers

For years, scientists have searched for a way to *completely* prevent sunburn. Skolex is the result of that search—the only preparation of its kind that assures you of complete safety from painful sunburn. Ask your druggist for Skolex Sun Allergy Cream today. (For a glorious tan—use Skol Suntan Lotion.)

---

*I*n ancient Greece, women counted their age from their wedding date. From 1950 to 1960, women got married at the youngest average age in recorded history: 20.3. (The average age for a first marriage in 1890 was 22.)

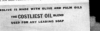

New Complexion Dial in Powder Room Pastels

PASTEL PINK

PASTEL BLUE

NEW GOLDEN DIAL

PASTEL GREEN

Contains a wondrous new Skin Freshener for better than ever protection under make-up!

Complexion Dial's gentle new Skin Freshener—Super AT-7—does what no ordinary soap, no drying synthetic, no greasy skin cream can possibly do! Sweeps away bacteria that so often spoil your complexion — without drying or greasing your skin!

Then, Complexion Dial's new Skin Freshener *stays on* your skin. You can't see it or feel it. But it's there, protecting the beauty of your complexion all day — even under make-up!

Today, buy Complexion Dial in colors — by the color of its gleaming new wrapper.

Match your tile with Dial!

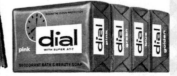

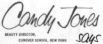

Candy Jones says

BEAUTY DIRECTOR,
CONOVER SCHOOL, NEW YORK

"Watch your skin thrive on Cashmere Bouquet Soap!"

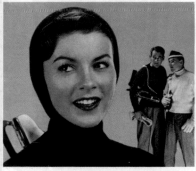

Winter sports play rough with your skin . . . but *you can* protect it. Cashmere Bouquet's 3-way beauty care does wonders for your skin!

Cleans cleaner than creams. Your skin is so much cleaner when you use Cashmere Bouquet! No cream film!

Stimulates with no astringent sting, when you stroke Cashmere Bouquet's mild lather into your skin.

Softens without lotion stickiness. Leaves normal, dry or oily skin naturally softer and smoother!

it gives your skin 3-way beauty care!

You can forget about greasy cleansing creams, sticky lotions, and stinging astringents! Because now, with just a cake of Cashmere Bouquet Soap, you can give your skin the beauty care of famous Conover students. This wonderful 3-way beauty care actually *cleans cleaner than creams . . . stimulates gently, softens and smooths your skin,* too. Just like using a whole row of beauty products . . . but so much quicker and easier. Start today and watch *your* skin thrive!

Cashmere Bouquet
TOILET SOAP

REGULAR
OR BIG BATH SIZE

---

*I*t's fairly common for famous folks to fib about their age; it's rumored that even Estée Lauder's family wasn't sure of her actual age when she passed away in 2004.

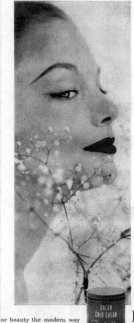

Not a half hearted liquid!
Not an oily heavy cream!
Not an 'all purpose' cream!

Salon Cold Cream

cleans cleaner because it has balanced emulsifying action!

Salon Cold Cream's special formula allows just the right amount of liquid to take its purifying oils deep down into your skin, there to melt and draw to the surface the old dirt, make-up and hardened secretions that block your pores.

You can be sure when you tissue it off that you are removing clogging impurities that could cause blemishes! Soap doesn't go deep enough to do it. Some liquid cleansers are too watery, others not effective enough to lift out deep-dirt. And oily, heavy creams do not have the emulsifying action needed to dislodge embedded grime.

See for yourself! Give your skin one deep cleansing with fluffy, silky Salon Cold Cream. Have the radiantly clean skin today that promises you clear, beautiful skin tomorrow. 3 ounces $1.25; 6 ounces $2.25.

Big plus: Salon Cold Cream leaves an invisible shield to help guard your skin against dryness!

In Canada, too.

or beauty the modern way

Dorothy Gray

44

The bluish-green color of Estée Lauder product packaging is actually known as "Estée Lauder Blue" or Pantone color 655. She chose this color for its muted elegance and because it complemented most bathroom décor.

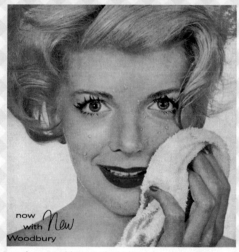

now New with Woodbury

wash natural beauty back into your complexion

EXCLUSIVE LOTION CONCENTRATE HELPS SKIN MOISTURIZE ITSELF!

Luxuriously different from today's drying toilet bars...fragrant new Woodbury is a facial beauty bar. Its unique ingredient—a beauty lotion concentrate— helps hold in your skin's own moisture to prevent dryness. Milder, creamier lather silkens your complexion...a gentle antiseptic combats blemishes.

Try this New Woodbury Beauty Facial. Work in rich lather with upward, outward motions. Rinse with warm water, then cold. Pat face with ice in soft cloth.

INTRODUCTORY OFFER:
Buy three bars, get a fourth for just 1¢.
Dream Pink or Spray Green.

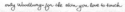

only Woodbury—for the skin you love to touch

Tan gloriously

Now get a lovelier, smoothe tan . . . faster . . . with Skol' exclusive formula

● You can be a sun-goddess with out a care . . . get the most strik ingly beautiful tan of your life, whe you smooth on marvelous new formula Skol. Two recent dermato logical discoveries—used only i Skol—scientifically screen out th rays that scorch and burn . . . filte in all the tanning rays to turn you skin a lovely, tawny tan.

This new Skol formula lets yo play in the sun hours longer—ta faster, more safely and comfortably Non-greasy, non-oily Skol doesn' pick up sand. Also in plastic bottles

Swimsuit by Catalina

SKOL

PROMOTES A BENEFICIAL TAN
PREVENTS PAINFUL SUNBURN
CONTAINS NO GREASE—NOT OILY

Used by more people than any other suntan 'lotion'

45

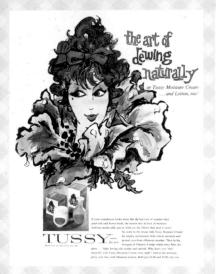

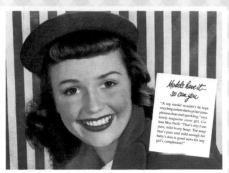

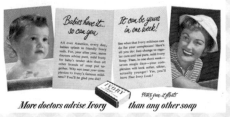

None of the three grande dames of modern cosmetics were born in America. Estée Lauder was born in Hungary, Helena Rubenstein was born in Poland, and Elizabeth Arden was born in Canada.

Albolene makeup remover, which is widely used to remove stage makeup, was actually developed by OB/GYNs to cleanse newborn babies.

KLEENEX® Tissues were actually invented as a hygienic way to remove cold cream.

the box caught my eye...
the tissue made me sigh...

Ah-h- **yes**

Hat by Mr. John

stronger!

more absorbent!

so lint-free!

Yes, there's a promise of something
finer in this box of frosty blue. And the
tissues . . . those soft, soft YES tissues . . .
more than make the promise good. Next time,
try YES. See and feel the difference.

Fluffy-soft YES tissues are stronger!
Downy-soft YES tissues are more absorbent!
Zephyr-soft YES tissues are so lint-free!

Chapter 2

Glamorous Cosmetics

✦✦✦◆ 🔲 ◆✦✦✦✦

In the 1940s, 1950s, and 1960s, cosmetic application was very much an art form, albeit a female dominated one. Abstract expressionist artists like Jackson Pollock or Willem de Kooning expressed themselves through spontaneity and kinetic painting techniques. For women of the same era, the art of artifice was a more subtle pursuit. Color and coif were likely chosen in as calculated a manner as the restrained but effusive bursts of color present in the artist Piet Mondrian's work.

Until the freedom of the mid 1960s, a woman's makeup application technique was frequently her main form of self-expression, and usually fashioned after her favorite celebrity. She could be slightly rebellious like Natalie Wood with her imperfect hair and tentative smile; she could expose her vulnerability by piling her hair atop her head like the waif-like Audrey Hepburn, or she could bleach her hair to a shade of Arctic blonde like the uber-cool Kim Novak.

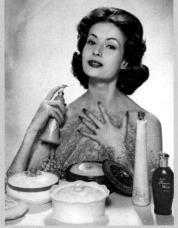

Women of the time were more a decoration for their husbands than an equal partner. Makeup offered an outlet to assert their control, personality, and aspirations. To that end, lipstick was both a statement and a form of power. A bold vermillion mouth expressed overt sexuality, while pink was more playful and girlish. In the era of society-girl-turned-princess Grace Kelly, cosmetics could express "High Society Summer" or a palette of "Royalty Red."

Cosmetics of the time were packaged ornate compacts and heavily-embellished cases. Much like their users, these products were meant to be displayed and shown off to friends. So enamored were women with their cosmetics that miniature symbols of makeup like tiny lipsticks or compacts were worn on charm bracelets.

Many modern-day cosmetic manufacturers and fashion designers cite this golden era of product design as their inspiration. Twins Jean and Jane Ford are the Patty Duke-like co-creators of Benefit Cosmetics. Their cheeky cosmetics include 1950s-inspired product names, glamorous powder puffs, and bodacious brand icons. "With beauty, you have to have a fabulous sense of humor," muses Jean. "Goldie Hawn captures that beauty. She is funny and smart, and that makes her even more beautiful."

Famed wit Dorothy Parker mentions humor, not lipstick, as part of her grooming routine. "The first thing I do in the morning is brush my teeth and sharpen my tongue." Lucille Ball was not only a comedic genius and consummate businesswoman, but also a celebrated beauty, and one of thirty actresses up for the role of Scarlett O'Hara in *Gone with the Wind*. But it was her self-deprecating wit that endured. For the majority of women of that era, though, brains and humor weren't the priority. It was beauty that closed the deal. Their gold-toned lipstick cases, decorated compacts, and ornate perfume bottles were their weapons of choice.

In 1962, three years before she took over the helm at *Cosmopolitan* magazine, Helen Gurley Brown penned a guide to life for single women of that era. *Sex and the Single Girl* included some solid advice, but in an era of standardized beauty and catch a man-centric advice, it also advised liberated women on what to cook for their men—both for the night before and the morning after. Forty years later, Candace Bushnell gave single women something to bond over with the television series *Sex and the City*. Has the message changed drastically in the intervening years? Not really. Bushnell's characters spend much of their existence primping, planning for, and re-hashing their flirtations and escapades with the opposite sex. The show's finale included a happily ever after moment worthy of a 1950s-era starlet.

No matter what the decade, feminine beauty and the tools of the trade play a starring role in the ritual of flirtation. Harvard Law Professor Doug Stone is a negotiation and communications specialist and the co-author of *Difficult Conversations*. Stone theorizes that using one's beauty and the accoutrements thereof, whether for flirting or negotiation, is frequently second nature. "Sometimes," he says, "our most natural instincts are those we're not aware of."

In the right circumstances the very act of applying makeup can be viewed as flirtation. While some beauty rituals are best kept secret, others become innately sensual when visible for public observation. Some women refuse to as much as tuck a stray hair aside in public, while others think nothing of applying a full face of makeup on the NYC subway system.

Beauty rituals, it seems, vary not only from decade to decade but from face to glamorous face.

Now...the first, luscious high-gloss lipstick!

'Lustrous' Lipstick

Designed for the smart woman...
who insists on that dewy look on her lips!

There's a special look a smart woman has that others always notice . . . a polished, shining look of utter elegance. You see it above all in her moist, radiant lips. Perhaps you've wished *you* could have this look . . . but never found the secret. Well, look no more. It's Revlon's 'Lustrous' Lipstick . . . the *extra-creamy* lipstick created to give your lips a

luscious, high-gloss glow . . . and brilliant color. Wear? Remarkably! Choose Revlon's 'Lustrous' to give your lips the soft, *dewy* look.

Also by Revlon . . . famous 'Lanolite' Lipstick . . . the only non-smear-type lipstick that stays on and on without drying your lips!

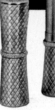

26 fabulous 'Lustrous' colors . . . in jeweler-designed 'Futurama' case. 1.35 to 37.50 plus tax.

© REVLON, INC. 1957

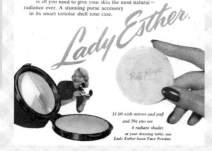
*P*rolonged eye contact, batting one's eyelashes, and winking were major flirting techniques in days gone by. In Japan it's considered rude to stare, and listeners focus on the speaker's neck (a practice started in Samurai times when peasants caught looking a samurai in the eye could be beheaded).

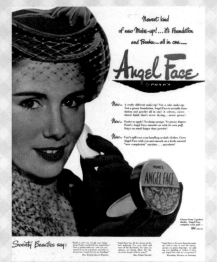

Newest kind of new Make-up!...it's Foundation and Powder...all in one—

Angel Face
by POND'S

New — A really different make-up! Not a color make-up. Not a greasy foundation. Angel Face is actually foundation and powder all in one! A velvety, sweettinted finish that's never drying...never greasy!

New — Easier to apply! No damp sponge. No greasy fingers. Pond's Angel Face smooths on with its own puff. Stays on much longer than powder!

New — Can't spill over your handbag or dark clothes. Carry Angel Face with you and smooth on a fresh, natural "new complexion" anytime...anywhere!

Choose from 5 perfect shades. Angel Face complete with puff—

Society Beauties say:

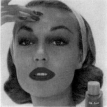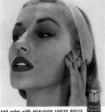

Helena Rubinstein tells you how to make up with silk!

Smooth on SILK-TONE* FOUNDATION. Helena Rubinstein, world-famous beauty authority, creates fluid silken make-up that covers every tiny line while it moisturizes with rich emollients. Apply dots of SILK-TONE to your cheeks, chin, nose, forehead—then spread evenly. In seven skin tones, 1.50.

Add color with SILK-TONE LIQUID ROUGE on a soft and satiny blend. A triangle of dots placed under the eyes (as shown above) and then blended quickly, will give you enough glorious glow to last all day long! SILK-TONE LIQUID ROUGE by Helena Rubinstein® comes in Coral, Red or Pink Tones, 1.25.

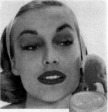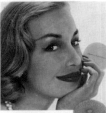

Puff on fine SILK-SCREEN FACE POWDER. Helena Rubinstein, color genius, blends this powder with atomized silk. Press on generously, then puff off excess to give you lasting, silken radiance. Ten shades, 1.25. Also ENGLISH COMPLEXION POWDER with imported silk, 3.50.

Touch up with SILKEN MINUTE MAKE-UP. It's a silken foundation and face powder all in one! Just puff it on as you would face powder. In a minute, you see a lovely silken radiance that clings for hours! Eight lively colors in a pretty purse compact, 1.25. *All prices plus federal tax.*

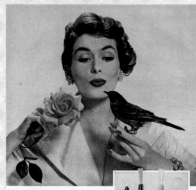

Robins and Roses...

are just around the corner . . . at the Cutex counter!

From Robin-Reds to Rosy Pinks—all the prettiest shades of spring are at your favorite toiletries counter! Select some sparkling new Cutex colors for your lips and fingertips today. Spring will seem a little sunnier if you do!

Why Pay More? Then invest new Cutex Chip-proof nail polish, with Enrichin, wears best...absolutely defies chipping!

The Most Kissable Lips Wear Cutex Lipstick! So long-lasting, it stays on hours longer—after eating, smoking, even kissing. Much creamier too, because Cutex Lipstick contains pure, SUPER LANOLIN. Keeps lips always soft as a rose!

Colors created courtesy DINAH ME-PINK SHADES and ROSE-PEARL colors

CUTEX

"*F*ire and Ice," one of Revlon's most popular lipstick shades ever, was marketed for either the naughty or nice part of a woman's personality. Accompanying advertising and product inserts featured a questionnaire to help women figure out which category they fell into.

52

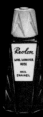

smart women everywhere

swear by *Revlon*

nail mamel 60¢
lipstick 60¢ also $1 size

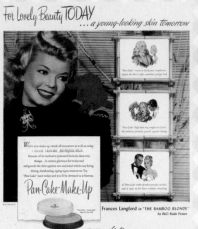
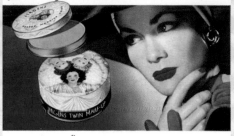
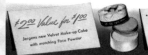
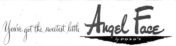
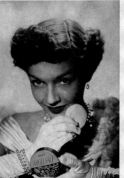
Tangee lipsticks ran an advertising campaign during the mid 1940s that praised women for doing a man's job, but who still looked feminine by wearing lipstick. Their ads paired concepts like beauty and liberty.

TAKE TIME OUT FOR BEAUTY

WHEN YOUR
AVON REPRESENTATIVE CALLS

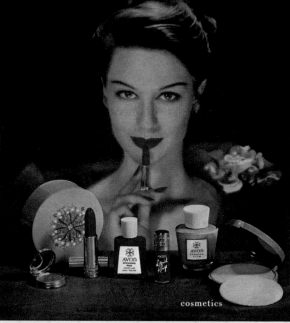

cosmetics

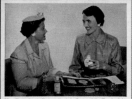

Mrs. Henry Lewis Ewan, wife of the Rector of the Church of the Transfiguration in Arcadia California, is shown (at right) taking time out to select Avon cosmetics with the help of Mrs. Virginia M. Duncan, her Avon Representative. Mrs. Ewan's church and P.T.A. activities keep her very busy, so she appreciates the convenience of shopping at home the Avon way.

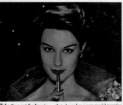

Take time out for beauty . . . that phrase has a very special meaning for the millions of women who select their cosmetics the Avon way. The wide and wonderful selection of Avon cosmetics and fragrances . . . the splendid assistance of your Avon Representative . . . the pleasingly moderate prices . . . are all reasons to take time out for beauty when your Avon Representative calls.

Your Avon Representative will be calling soon . . . Welcome her!

IF YOU WISH AN AVON REPRESENTATIVE TO CALL, PLEASE CONSULT YOUR
LOCAL PHONE DIRECTORY OR CALL WESTERN UNION OPERATOR 25

Avon cosmetics
RADIO CITY, NEW YORK

---

*S*ongs with "lipstick" in the titles include: "Lipstick, Powder, and Paint" by Big Joe Turner, "Mystic Lipstick" by Christy Moore, "I Hate Your Lipstick" by Veal, "Lipstick on Your Collar" by Connie Francis, and "Lucky Lipstick" by Surferosa.

based on his make-up research for color TV

Max Factor creates

a new kind of lipstick!

new! the color won't come off until you take it off!

new! no waiting for it to set! no blotting!

new! it never, never dries your lips!

new! the brilliant beauty of high fidelity colors!

Max Factor's **hi-fi** Lipstick

Now... at the price of ordinary lipstick...Revlon *gives you the magnificent luxury of 'Futurama'!*

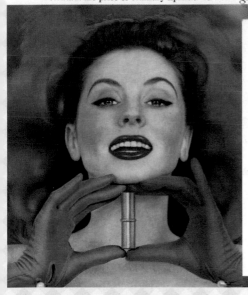

Revlon's new
fabulous 'Futurama' case
with lipstick refill– only 1.25!

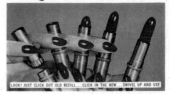

LOOK! JUST CLICK OUT OLD REFILL ... CLICK IN THE NEW ... SWIVEL UP AND USE

Your jeweler-designed 'Futurama' case goes on forever—all you ever buy again are Revlon refills! You save 35¢ on every lipstick!

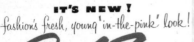

IT'S NEW !
fashion's fresh, young 'in-the-pink' look!

Angel Face
BY POND'S

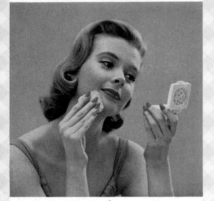

IT'S NEW ! the adorable pink
Date Case

Newest way to carry your heavenly new complexion

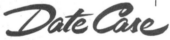

Who's the girl with the Angel Face?

Is she young? Sweet? *Naturally* pretty?
Yes! With one quick touch of Angel Face!
Is her face velvety *smooth?* Never shiny, never dry?
Of course! She'd never dream of using greasy make-ups or drying cake powders!
Does she look fresh and aglow—after hours and hours?
Naturally. Her Angel Face by Pond's clings, because it's a magical blend of finest powder and smoothing vaporized beauty oils!

Could be this "Angel Face" is you! More girls do use Pond's Angel Face than any other make-up! In 3 luscious fashion pinks—Blushing Angel, Pink Angel, Blonde Angel. And 5 other heavenly shades. All in the new pink "Date Case!"

The new "Date" Case, with mirror and puff, only 79¢, plus tax.

Today's most popular make-up—by far!

Slow down—this is a red you have to see! A bright, blazing, stop-and-look red...hard to miss, but awfully easy to wear. For Look-Out Red is *all* red —no trace of orange or blue—and perfect with every stitch you own. It's a Cashmere Bouquet red that stays red and stays on—hour after hour!

7 Cover-Girl Colors 49¢ *plus tax*

cashmere bouquet
INDELIBLE-TYPE LIPSTICK
Super-creamed to Keep Your Lips Like Velvet

Conover Girls Pick Cashmere Bouquet!

Advice from the Beauty Director of the Conover School: "Use a lip brush for a sharp, clear outline. Then fill in with short, slant strokes of your Cashmere Bouquet lipstick."

Candy Jones

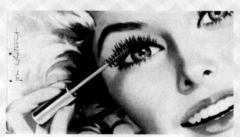

New, really waterproof
"MAGIC" MASCARA
by Maybelline only $1

No more stuck-together lashes! No more stiff, coated-look or feel. New *Spiral Brush* separates lash-by-lash as it colors and curls. Automatically applies just enough color around each lash individually. Far better than a rod! And smudge-proof "MAGIC" formula is *really* waterproof, yet completely gentle. No sting, no odor.

Maybelline—always the purest and best in eye beauty

Lasts for months

REFILLS 69¢

*D*uring World War II the War Production Board tried to restrict production of cosmetics since it believed that the materials used to create these cosmetics would better serve the war effort. While women were willing to give up most of their makeup, they generally refused to part with their lipstick.

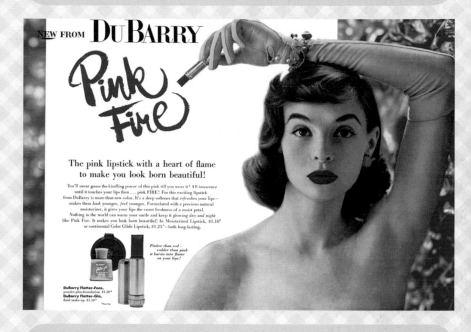

*D*ifferent body parts are used to describe emotions. Cheek, cheeky— means being fresh or rude (sometimes in a good way). Lip, mouth off—talking back to, being disrespectful. Eye—checking out, giving the once over to.

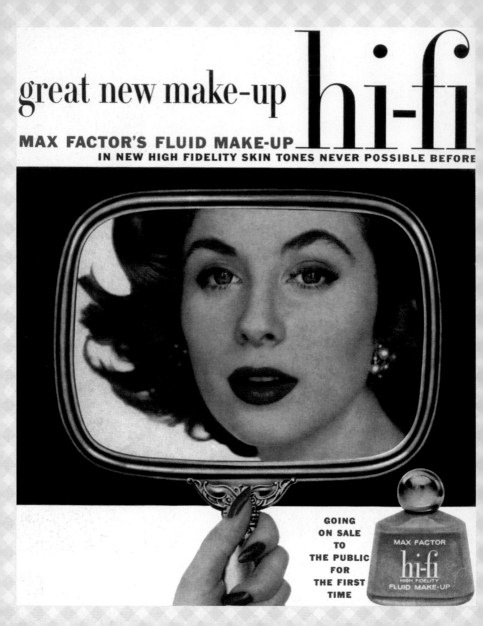

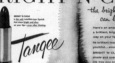

A recent survey found that 72 percent of people perceive those who smile often to be more self-assured and successful, while 86 percent are more likely to flirt with strangers if they are smiling.

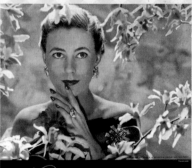

During World War II it was considered patriotic to wear bright red lipstick.

Louis Philippe

Where else would an eye for beauty end its search! Here are colors that captivate...Louis Philippe shades of fashion matched in lipstick and rouge. And to complete the allure, lovely ladies smooth on Louis Philippe cake make-up with devastating effect!

Lipstick creme base of satin sheen and incredible clinging power. 9 luscious shades. *Rouge* creme or dry, to match. *Cake make-up* with the creme-y base that protects as it beautifies. 6 harmonizing shades. At cosmetic counters everywhere.

THIS SPRING HE'LL *Love you in Pink!*

NEW *Pink'n Sassy*
A gay, party-going pink—feminine as it is fiery! Wear it when you're in the mood for spur-of-the-moment dates . . . lively teasin . . . a sudden kiss!

NEW *Pink'n Sweet*
Pink for a proposal! Marriage on your mind? This is for you . . . a tempting, rosy-soft pink . . . so romantic, it's practically guaranteed to make it happen!

Stroke Me Pink... dramatic, sophisticated! For the moments when you feel very "femme fatale" . . . in the mood for a Paris hat . . . a new love affair!

CUTEX

puts your love-life in the pink with the prettiest shades of the season! Try some of this Cutex color-magic tonight . . . and listen for those sure-to-be-whispered words . . . "LOVE YOU IN PINK"!

*L*eonardo da Vinci invented the concept of contact lenses in 1508 when he sketched corrective lenses to be applied directly to the eye. French philosopher René Descartes came up with his own version in 1636, but it wasn't until the nineteenth century that Adolf Fick developed glass contact lenses.

RIDESCENT MAGIC
new luminous lipstick brings them excitingly alive with soft shimmering beauty

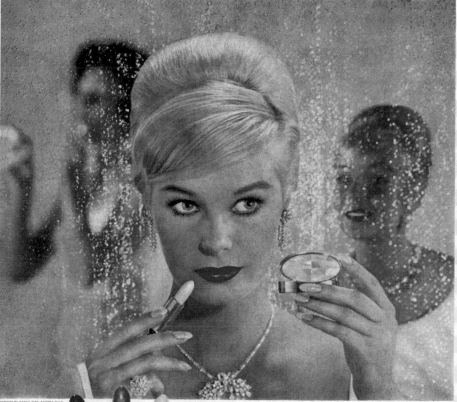

PETAL FROST · FLAMINGO PEARL · ORCHID PEARL · DESERT PEARL · ESSENCE OF PEARL · APRICOT FROST · GOLDEN FROST

IT'S NEW! IT'S DAZZLING! It's different from any lipstick you've ever known! These are truly iridescent lipcolors that gleam with silver through and through. Only from MAX FACTOR at $1.25*...each fits the glamorous HI-SOCIETY mirror-cases.

new Film-Finish Face Powter

– finest texture ever loveliest shades . . . for that exciting Hollywood "finish"

Inspired by Hollywood! Designed to make you look as the stars look on the screen. A new . . . *really new* powder . . . but already thousands of happy girls have found the enchantment of skin-glamour through Woodbury Film-Finish Powder!

A 5-stage blending process produces the *loveliest-ever shades* that really stay lovely on your skin . . . *smoothest-ever texture* that clings longer . . . hides beauty-marring blemishes and lines far better than ever.

Film-Finish never clogs, cakes, turns pasty . . . never makes your skin look "porey". But fluff on some this very night and let your man prove what it does for you. 8 shades, including midsummer magic colors.

Lucille Ball
in
Metro-Goldwyn-Mayer's
Technicolor Hit
"ZIEGFELD FOLLIES"

Woodbury SUN PEACH, midsummer-dream enchantment for a sun-kissed skin like Lucille Ball's . . . and yours.

Choose your own Star-Styled Shade for a Date-Success Summer

SUN-KISSED SKIN? SUN PEACH, Lucille Ball's shade . . . *star-radiance for sun-kissed skin!*

BRUNETTE, Ava Gardner's shade . . . *exciting warmth for pale dark skin!*

MEDIUM SKIN? WINDSOR ROSE, Shirley Temple's shade . . . *fresh rose prettiness for pink-toned medium skin!*

CHAMPAGNE RACHEL, Susan Peters' shade . . . *golden drama for honey-toned skin!*

FAIR SKIN? NATURAL, Gloria De Haven's shade: *flower-fairness for pink-and-white skin!*

RACHEL, Hedy Lamarr's shade . . . *creamy enchantment for pale ivory skin!*

SUMMERTIME MATCHED MAKE-UP $1. Matching lipstick and rouge at no extra cost with the big box of Woodbury Powder! Get your summer-success glamour trio, now! No change in the box; all Woodbury Powder now on sale is the new "Film-Finish".

Also boxes of Woodbury Powder, 25¢ and 10¢, plus tax.

Woodbury
FILM-FINISH
Powder

Helena Rubinstein Announces
New Silk Powder and Foundation

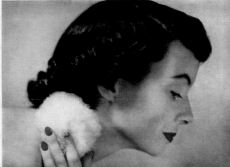

Blended with pure *SILK*...to give you the "Silken Look"

Who would dream of blending silk—gossamer silk—into foundation and face powder? Only Helena Rubinstein, the world's leading beauty authority!

Silk Foundations smooth your skin to new texture perfection, impart new color vibrancy, protect and beautify for hours on end.

Silk Screen Face Powder sheers on more delicately, imparts exquisite young bloom and clings longer—with silken magnetism.

Let it be the "Silken Look" for your own

gala holiday season—and give it to every woman on your Christmas list.

Silk Screen Face Powder	$1.00
Silk Compact Powder, compressed	1.00
Silk-Film, cream-water foundation	1.25
Silk-Tone, creamy liquid foundation	1.50
Gift box—powder, lipstick, rouge	3.00
All in harmonizing skin tones	

For expert advice on how to apply make-up write today for Helena Rubinstein's free 16-page illustrated booklet "Make-Up Palette."

---

*T*he director D. W. Griffith is credited for inventing the first false eyelashes, worn by an actress in his 1916 film *Intolerance*. It wasn't until the mid 1960s that false eyelashes became really popular, when designer Mary Quant declared them to be a must-have beauty accessory.

---

double dare red

Throw caution to the winds! Wear Avon's thrilling Double Dare Red on your lips and finger tips. It's a challenge in color... intriguingly packaged to double dare you to look your loveliest.

Your Avon Representative will bring it directly to your home.

Welcome her when she calls.

Avon
cosmetics
AT RADIO CITY · NEW YORK

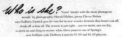

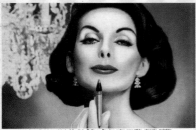

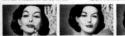

These fishy facts about lipstick might really bug you. Pearl Essence, which adds a sexy shimmer to many lipstick brands, is derived from fish scales, mainly herring. Carmine, a red dye used in the production of lipstick, is made from the crushed shells of the female cochineal beetle.

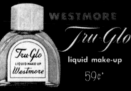

Fresh...young...alive! Here's the look you've been looking for

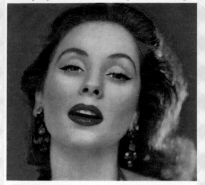

Now! Give your skin tone the color lift it needs with

Revlon 'Touch-and-Glow'
The Liquid Make-Up

Here is your glow . . . loveliest of all . . . a fragile, sheltered look that's, oh, so naturally feminine! Revlon 'Touch-and-Glow' is a delicate touch—never cakey, never drying. Every drop of this moisturizing liquid make-up is blended with Revlon's precious Lanolin to pamper your skin— keep it dewy-fresh. So just touch . . . and glow! You've found the look you've been looking for! Nobody knows you wear it but you!

Now in 9 living shades, 1.25 and 1.75 plus tax
Face powder in harmonies, 1.25 • .s. tax

It's new! It's wonderful!
It doesn't spill . . . it doesn't make
. . . it doesn't crumble . . . yet it powders
at the feather-touch of a puff

YARDLEY
Feather-Pressed
powder

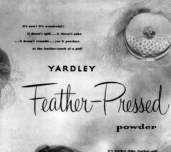

It's feather-light, feather-soft,
feather-smooth face powder in its
own handy, purse-perfect compact . . .
compact, $3.75; refill, in its own
portable case, with puff, $1. both plus tax

PINK
A
BOO

A playful pink . . . but it's strictly for grown-ups! There's nothing little-girl about the kiss-me-quick look it gives your lips. This bright new shade of Cashmere Bouquet Lipstick does its good work discreetly, too— *Pink-A-Boo* stays on *you*, stays off everyone else!

7 Cover-Girl Colors **49¢** plus tax

**Conover
girls pick
Cashmere
Bouquet**

"Have a lipstick wardrobe: a blue-red, an orange-red and a definite pink. All three cost less than $2 when, like our Conover girls, you choose Cashmere Bouquet".

Candy Jones

cashmere bouquet
Indelible-Type Lipstick
Super-Creamed to Keep Your Lips Like Velvet

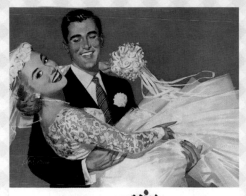

...and from this day forward, _ever-lovin'_ **viv**

the lipstick that stays married to your lips

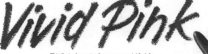

Vivid Pink

This Spring's prettier-than-ever, ever-vivid pink

A decidedly new kind of Pink . . . a fun lovin', fun-to-wear VIVID PINK promising rich, deeply glowing color that no other lipstick can ever hope to match. You know this color won't forsake you, won't stray, won't fade . . . for this is the one-and-only, ever-true, ever-lovin' viv and it's made by Toni.

VIV REGULAR
creamy non-smear type $1.50 plus tax

VIV SUPER LIPSTICK
new 24-hour lipstick $1.25 plus tax

in 12 vivid springtime shades

drive plus tax

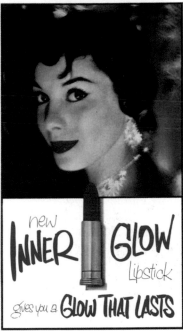

at last! all-day color that **WON'T GO FLAT**

new **INNER GLOW** _Lipstick_

gives you a **GLOW THAT LASTS**

At last an all-day lipstick that just won't get that flat look—a lipstick that stays fresh and glowing even when it's been on all day. Fabulous new INNER GLOW lipstick glows on and on—with soft, shimmering color! INNER GLOW actually puts a dew-soft, transparent color-guard on your lips! It's the new secret of lips that stay velvety-soft and moist—of radiance that lasts without a letdown all the livelong day! **79¢** PLUS TAX

7 INNER GLOW COLORS

RHYTHM-IN-RED—blue-red
PINK PLUM—deep pink
LOOK-OUT RED—true-red
PINK-A-BOO—rosy pink
TROPIC SUN—golden red
PEACH-OF-A-PINK—rosy coral
CORAL—bright coral

CASHMERE BOUQUET COSMETICS... _for all your beauty needs_

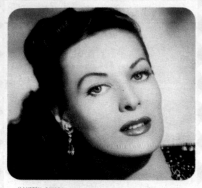

MAUREEN O'HARA starring in Universal-International's LADY GODIVA
PRINT BY TECHNICOLOR

Glorifying drops
beautify your complexion instantly!

HOLLYWOOD'S famous make-up artists, Westmore Brothers, have created a complexion miracle for movie stars — and you. A few glorifying, concealing, creamy drops of TRU-GLO on your chin, forehead and each cheek — blended in with fingertips — and your skin is instantly smoother, lovelier! For all types of skin; many shades. *Guaranteed no finer quality at any price.* At all variety and drug stores.

59¢*

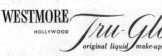

WESTMORE *Tru-Glo*
HOLLYWOOD
original liquid make-up

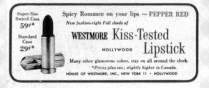

Super-Size Swivel Case 59¢*

Standard Case 29¢*

Spicy Romance on your lips — PEPPER RED
New fashion-right Fall shade of

WESTMORE **Kiss-Tested** Lipstick
HOLLYWOOD

Many other glamorous colors, stay on all around the clock.
*Prices plus tax; slightly higher in Canada.
HOUSE OF WESTMORE, INC., NEW YORK 11 • HOLLYWOOD

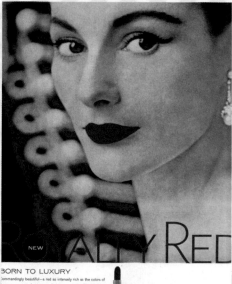

NEW

LADY RED

BORN TO LUXURY

Commandingly beautiful—a red as intensely rich as the colors of the new season's fashions—soft, lustrous, elegant. Royalty Red was created to make you, and everything you wear, important. Royalty Red is a *Sheer Velvet Lipstick*—in creamy or stay-all-day types—and magnificent new refill cases. $1.35, $2.00.

For beauty the modern way . . .
Dorothy Gray

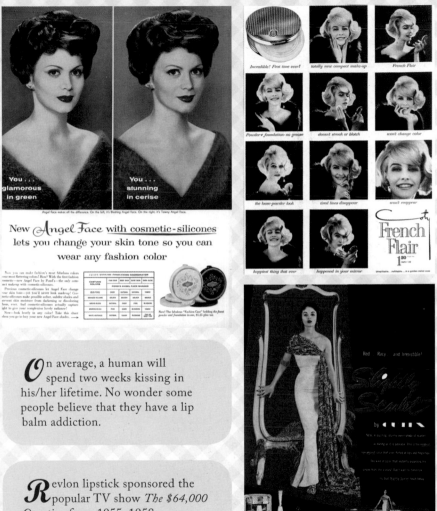

On average, a human will spend two weeks kissing in his/her lifetime. No wonder some people believe that they have a lip balm addiction.

Revlon lipstick sponsored the popular TV show *The $64,000 Question* from 1955–1958.

71

NOW YOU CAN ERASE DARK CIRCLES— SHADOWS— BLEMISHES

WITH *erace*

THE ORIGINAL "COVER-UP" USED BEFORE MAKE-UP

Screen-TV secret released to the public for the first time
by **MAX FACTOR** World's foremost make-up authority

HERE IS THE "MIRACLE" YOU'VE BEEN HEARING ABOUT. At last, America's make-up authority, Max Factor, has released the secret substance he created to hide imperfections, lines, shadows and blemishes from the merciless scrutiny of motion picture and television cameras. Of all the many exclusive creations for which the "glamour industries" are indebted to Max Factor, this product is probably the one its beauties rely on most, day by day, to stay lovely.

And now this very product, ERACE, is available to you in a new form as simple to use as a lipstick.

SWIFTLY, INSTANTLY, every trace of "problem-points" which mar your beauty can disappear from sight. You're only seconds away from a flawless complexion with ERACE. In no way does ERACE alter the methods of beautification or make-up which you have found to be best for you. For ERACE is not a cosmetic . . . you use ERACE only *where it is needed, before* applying make-up or *without any make-up.*

AND HERE'S ANOTHER important fact we can't evade. From time to time every woman is subject to one of the "problems" ERACE was specifically created to overcome. Teenagers seem to "blossom forth" with blemishes just before that all-important "date". The passing years, loss of sleep or temporary physical indisposition will put ugly circles under the loveliest eyes . . . harsh lines in the smoothest complexion. For these problems and dozens more . . . ERACE is the answer.

TEST ERACE FOR YOURSELF
In the privacy of your own home, make this test . . . AT NO EXPENSE TO YOU!

1. Get ERACE today.
2. Apply to a shadow under just one eye . . . or a deep line on *one* side of your face.
3. Now . . . hold a mirror at arm's length. Look first at one side of your face . . . then the other. SEE THE AMAZING DIFFERENCE YOUR MIRROR DISCLOSES!

ONCE YOU HAVE MADE THIS TEST you will be *thrilled* with the difference, overwhelmed at the startling comparison . . . you will agree that you have at last found the answer to dark circles, shadows, blemishes . . . OR YOUR MONEY WILL BE REFUNDED!

ERACE BLENDS PERFECTLY
Regardless of your complexion "type", one of these exclusive Max Factor blending tones will match your coloring – Fair, Natural, Medium, Deep Natural, Tan, Deep Tan.

You'll find ERACE . . . this wonderfully easy to use, effective cover up . . . complete with instruction booklet in this attractive counter display.

LOOK FOR IT . . . TODAY!
Available now at your favorite drug and department store.

$1.75

ERACE—BY MAX FACTOR
the "cover-up" used *before* make-up

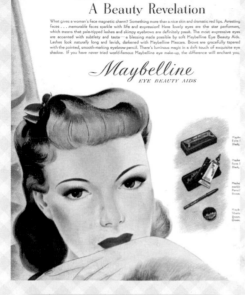

A Beauty Revelation

What gives a woman's face magnetic charm? Something more than a nice skin and dramatic red lips. Arresting faces . . . memorable faces sparkle with life and expression! Here lovely eyes are the star performers, which means that pale-tipped lashes and skimpy eyebrows are definitely passé. The most expressive eyes are accented with subtlety and taste—a blessing made possible by soft Maybelline Eye Beauty Aids. Lashes look naturally long and lavish, darkened with Maybelline Mascara. Brows are gracefully tapered with the pointed, smooth-marking eyebrow pencil. There's luminous magic in a soft touch of exquisite eye shadow. If you have never tried world-famous Maybelline eye make-up, the difference will enchant you.

Maybelline
EYE BEAUTY AIDS

a common urban myth is that the average woman consumes 6 pounds of lipstick in her lifetime. That would amount to noshing on about 95 tubes over a lifetime. (Guess that would explain the popularity of flavored lip gloss.)

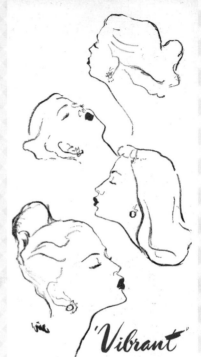

'Vibrant'

PARIS-BORN COLOR

It's the exciting new lip-look . . . clear, bright and lustrous . . . in smooth, smooth 'Sub-Deb' Lipstick. 'Vibrant' is one of eleven flattering Coty lipstick shades. And, to keep you picture-perfect, it is color-matched in 'Air-Spun' Face Powder and 'Sub-Tint' Cream-Powder Base. $1. *(plus tax)*

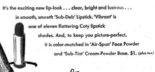

Coty 'SUB-DEB' LIPSTICK

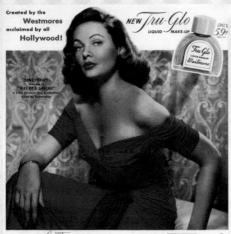
> *I*n the U.K. "slap" is another word for "makeup," from "slap up," a theatrical term for applying makeup. (Not to be confused with "slapper," which means a sexually promiscuous woman.)

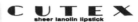

The original "sweater girl," Lana Turner, or rather Julia Jean Mildred Frances Turner, was discovered while drinking a soda pop at Schwab's Drugstore on Sunset Boulevard.

NEW! MAGNET RED

LIGHT

DAHLIA

GITANE

BALI

Enter with Flying Colors

See how stunningly Coty uses color ... to smarten both your lips and costume. Take Magnet Red.

Very new — it's very red. A dashing red, the make-up accent that your somber fall frocks need. Eight other high-fashion Coty shades offer an exciting choice. There's even a choice in cases. Newest is double "Sub-Deb," $1, more than double the size of regular "Sub-Deb" but only double the price. "Periscope" — the one-finger automatic style is available in five smart case colors, at $1.

Magnet Red" is available in the double "Sub-Deb" case. For all other shades, choose any case you like!

Coty

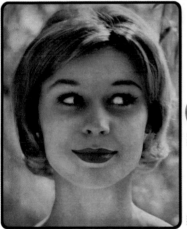

new!
"Satina Look" Compact translucent violet colored, holds Sheer Velvet pressed powder plus creamy foundation $2.50. Pay-it refill, 75c.

new!
Sheer Velvet Film, flattering liquid-oil foundation with amazing new moisturizing ingredient, $1.25

Most natural beauty in the history of make-up
...created with new Sheer Velvet

Now softly-radiant formula ... light, yet clinging and moisturized to give your skin a dewy, youthful look. Covers imperfections to perfection. Looks completely natural, even in morning sunlight ... stays fresh all day and prevents that mid-afternoon tired look. Start with Sheer Velvet Film, the ideal make-up foundation. Touch up as needed through the day with Sheer Velvet Compact. Both in 6 lustrous shades.

Dorothy Gray

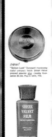

she's got viv

(you can have it, too!)

It's not so much beauty as it is personal vibrancy and sparkle, and all those indefinable qualities that make everyone instantly aware of her.

For sure there's a new lipstick that brings out all the vividness and sparkle of the real you with exciting colors that make you look and feel vividly alive. It's the new VIV lipstick by Tintl. VIV's new High-Chroma Formula gives you the most vivid colors any woman has ever worn. Choose from six bright shades, each as sparkling as the Vivid Coral you see here. Try VIV, that vivid new lipstick by Tintl.

Comfortable, long-lasting and very, very vivid.

new viv lipstick by Tintl

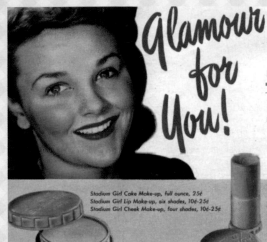

Glamour for You!

There's a new thrill waiting for you... a fresh, captivating complexion!

With Stadium Girl Cake Make-up your complexion appears lovelier, more romantic than ever...a truly enchanting skin beauty that remains soft and natural for hours. Then, too, remember Stadium Girl Cake Make-up hides those tiny, annoying skin faults and brings about an overall complexion of warm overtones —thrillingly glamorous.

Try this sensational, new cake make-up. You'll find new glamour in one of these flattering shades—Natural, Rachel, Brunette, Golden Tan.

The modern plastic, waterproof Stadium Girl case makes a beautiful purse accessory. You'll want to carry it with you at all times.

Wherever you find Stadium Girl Cake Make-up, you'll find these other equally fine cosmetics—Stadium Girl Lip Make-up, Stadium Girl Cheek Make-up.

Stadium Girl Cake Make-up, full ounce, 25¢
Stadium Girl Lip Make-up, six shades, 10¢-25¢
Stadium Girl Cheek Make-up, four shades, 10¢-25¢

Available at 5¢ and 10¢ stores

Stadium Girl

CAMPUS SALES CO., Distributors
Milwaukee 2, Wis.

---

only AVON brings this COLOR MAGIC to you in your home

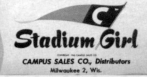

Coral...Nectar...Clear Red...Pink Cheer...Copper...
shades as fresh and new as spring in Avon Lipsticks and Matching Nail Polish

To complement your very own coloring, and give spring and summer costumes the just-right accent that makes you sparkle, Avon brings you this color enchantment!

You'll be thrilled by the soft, velvety texture of Avon Lipsticks ... the lasting smoothness of Super-Creamy ... the luxury-long flattery of Avon's new Color-Last Lipstick. And you'll like the note of perfection achieved by wearing nail polish in an exactly matching shade. (There are twelve shades in all.) Like thousands of other smart women, you will delight in the soothing creams, softening lotions and the other aids to good grooming which Avon alone can bring to you in your home. The next or your family will like your choosing economy-wise Avon Toiletries for them, too!

The Avon way of buying cosmetics is such a pleasant, personal one. You select them in your home from your Avon Representative. The cosmetics and toiletries correct for your complexion needs are easy to choose, with her helpful guidance, from Avon's wide and wonderful selection.

...Welcome her when she calls

Your Avon Representative helps you choose cosmetics best suited to your needs

You'll find it so easy and pleasant to shop the Avon way ... right in your own home. Your friendly Avon Representative helps you select cosmetics best for your own skin needs. At the same time, you can choose fine quality Avon toiletries for your whole family.

To obtain this service, simply call Western Union by number. Ask for Operator 25 and tell her you want to see an Avon Representative. Or, where this service is not available, please write directly to Avon at one of the addresses below.

THE BETTER KNOW OPERATOR 25 FOR YOUR AVON REPRESENTATIVE

Mrs. Dorothy Cameron, 911 North Street, Raleigh, North Carolina, Woman's Editor of Carolina's largest newspaper, seeks cosmetics in her home with the help of her AVON Representative, Mrs. Eileen Horne.

Avon cosmetics

MADE IN NEW YORK · PASADENA CALIFORNIA · MONTREAL CANADA

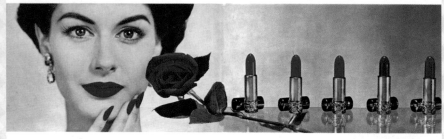

76

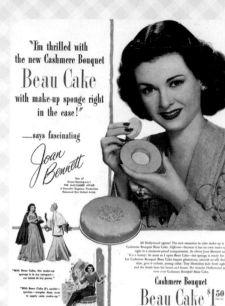

"I'm thrilled with the new Cashmere Bouquet **Beau Cake** with make-up sponge right in the case!"

—says fascinating *Joan Bennett*

Star of Ernest Hemingway's THE MACOMBER AFFAIR A Benedict Bogeaus Production Released thru United Artists

All Hollywood agrees! The new sensation in cake make-up is Cashmere Bouquet Beau Cake. *Different*—because it has its own make-up sponge right in a moisture-proof compartment. As clever Joan Bennett says:

"It's a beauty! As soon as I open Beau Cake—the sponge is ready for action." Let Cashmere Bouquet Beau Cake impart glamorous, smooth-as-silk finish to *your* skin; give it radiant, young color. Tiny blemishes fade from sight, and the finish lasts for hours and hours. No wonder Hollywood stars now trust Cashmere Bouquet Beau Cake.

"With Beau Cake, the make-up sponge is in my compact—not lost in my purse."

"With Beau Cake it's easier—quicker—simpler than ever to apply cake make-up."

Cashmere Bouquet Beau Cake $1⁵⁰

Gay new cake make-up with sponge compartment right in the case

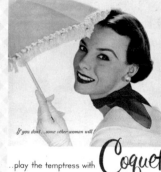

MAX FACTOR makes it a Hi-Society summer

Luscious lilting lipstick shades in colorful carefree cases. You'll love Hi-Society...dainty case, mirror, lipstick all-in-one. Complete with refill only $1.50.

GOLDEN ORANGE Lipstick Joyous sunlit shade, shown in a Gay Orange case. Happy complement for the new "off-white to beige" look.

PINK JADE Lipstick Orient's most precious color, shown in a Frosted White case. Ideal accent for summer tones. Also in Party-Pink case.

DAZZLING CORAL Lipstick To the light your lips, shown in a new Cool Blue case. Dainty accessory for the popular mauve to blue fashions.

The University of Illinois at Urbana–Champaign once had an Anti Lipstick Society. The men who belonged to the group were against heavy lipstick worn by women, and their motto was "Lips that touch lipstick shall never touch mine."

If you don't...some other woman will!

..play the temptress with *Coquette*

woodbury's fate-tempting powder color

Don't pretend you aren't making a play for him, little Coquette! You chose that flirtatious parasol. You made your complexion that tantalizing, tempting thing! For "Coquette" is the delicious, delightful, golden social powder shade for your skin...that the sun like best!

It's Woodbury, of course,...the powder with the unique ingredient that gives your skin the fabulous satin touch! Plus the clingability and cooked-flower fragrance that lingers for many romantic hours. Try Woodbury today! See the wonderful difference! 24c, 50c, $1.00 plus tax.

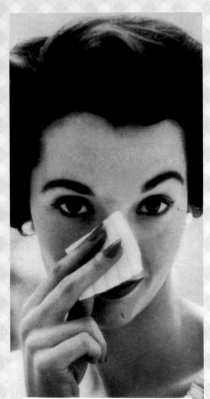

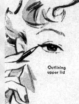

3 quick tricks to eye beauty

Outlining
upper lid

❶ With Maybelline soft Eyebrow Pencil, draw narrow line across upper eyelids, at base of lashes, adding short up-stroke at outer corner. Soften line with fingertip.

❷ Next, use short, light upward strokes of the Maybelline Eyebrow Pencil, to form beautiful, expressive brows. Taper lightly at outer end. Soften effect with fingertip.

Accenting
eyebrows

❸ Apply smooth Maybelline Mascara from base to tips of lashes, brushing upward. (Hold a few seconds to set "up-swoop.") For an extra touch of mysterious eye beauty blend a bit of Maybelline Eye Shadow on upper lid.

The world's smartest women depend on Maybelline soft eye make-up for heart-stirring beauty. Today, let Maybelline magic bring out the unsuspected loveliness of *your* eyes!

Maybelline

Mascara (plus
Eye Shadow)

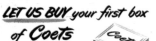
Maybelline mascara, originally made by chemist T. L. Williams out of Vaseline and coal dust, helped his sister Mabel attract her boyfriend. The name Maybelline is a portmanteau of Mabel and Vaseline.

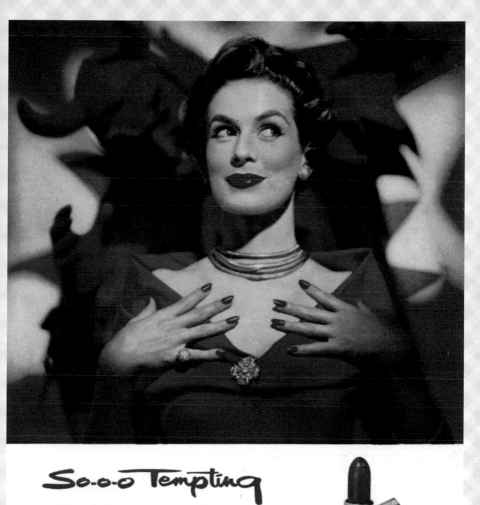

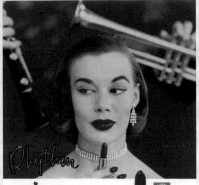

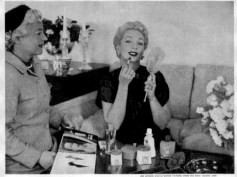

Rhythm in Red!

cashmere bouquet

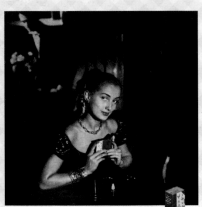

... the Mystery of the Beautiful Lady

PEGGY SAGE

In 1960, Elizabeth Taylor won an Academy Award for her portrayal of a prostitute in *Butterfield 8*. It's widely believed that the recently ill Taylor won the sympathy of the judges. Nominee Shirley MacLaine was said to have mournfully declared, "I lost to a tracheotomy!"

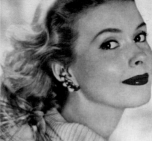

Helena Rubinstein

*E*gyptian queen Cleopatra wore kohl, eyeliner made from ground-up minerals. Elizabeth Taylor portrayed Cleopatra in the film version, which inspired a trend for heavily made-up eyes.

New <u>Silk-Tone</u> Liquid Make-Up gives instant radiance—all-day glamour!

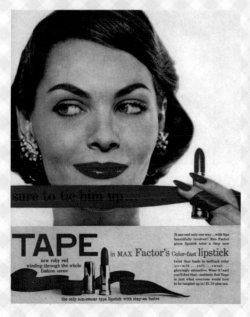

sure to tie him up ...

TAPE in MAX Factor's Color-fast lipstick

new ruby red
winding through the whole
fashion scene

It can end only one way...with lips beautifully involved! Max Factor gives lipstick color a deep new twist that leads to brilliant ruby wormth...soft...sweet...glowingly attractive. Wear it! and you'll find that—suddenly Red Tape is just what everyone would love to be tangled up in! $1.30 plus tax.

the only non-smear type lipstick with stay-on lustre

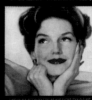

1st AUTOMATIC MASCARA WITH SELF-COATING APPLICATOR

NEW! BEAUTI-LASH

FOR BEAUTY THE MODERN WAY *Dorothy Gray*

Chapter 3
Lustrous, Lovely Locks
⬥⬦⬥⬦ ◧ ⬦⬥⬦⬥

Hair tends to take on mythical properties in legends, fairy tales, and Hollywood. When Rapunzel was locked away in her tower, her prince climbed her long golden tresses, thereby rescuing her from a future of spinsterhood *and* endless bad hair days. Lady Godiva's yards of hair saved her modesty on that long, nude horseback ride.

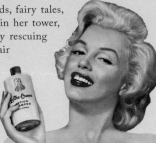

Marilyn Monroe was just plain Norma Jean, until she started a serious relationship with a bottle of peroxide. Rita Hayworth endured hours of painful electrolysis on her hairline to transform her from hirsute Margarita Carmen Cansino to sleek screen goddess Gilda. Veronica Lake may be the only starlet on public record who had the War Department request that she opt for a new 'do. During World War II, women everywhere copied her trademark "peek-a-boo" hairstyle, which consisted of long blonde waves covering one eye. Her look was sexy, but highly impractical for factory workers whose hair kept getting caught in the machinery. Talk about suffering for beauty.

In the early 1940s and through the war women's hairstyles were shorter and more practical, but by the end of the decade hair was longer and more glamorous. Snoods, hairnets, ribbons, and even turbans (yikes!) were commonplace accessories. In our own times we understand the serious psychological pain of a bad hair day. Back then, they'd just cover the embarrassing evidence with a fabulous fedora.

Leslie Caron and Audrey Hepburn playfully embodied the gamine look of the early 1950s, with sleekly cropped hair paired with hoop earrings. In the 1950s women went curl crazy and wore their hair waved, coiled, and crimped. Lucille Ball was the poster girl for the unfortunately named "poodle cut," while Grace Kelly and Sandra Dee embodied the more subtle variations on curl. Young girls wore their hair pulled back in ponytails and tied with frothy scarves. Their mothers were addicted to pin curls and home permanents—the revolutionary new way to smell up a Saturday afternoon. Rayve Wave promised "a softer, shinier, more natural curl!" and Lilt home permanent was the product that "you just squeeze on and love twice."

Color was paramount. "Does she… or doesn't she?" was the somewhat sly, somewhat smutty question on everyone's lips. But only her hairdresser knew for sure. New formulations ensured more subtle variations, so hair hue was no longer limited to Cleopatra charcoal or Marilyn platinum.

Conair was founded in 1959, and later introduced the first portable blowdryer, ensuring that henceforth women could endure hours of follicle distress in the comfort of their own homes. And then came the beehive and its love child, the bouffant. Those high-maintenance hairdos required stressful backcombing, teasing, and hair spraying. "The higher the hair, the closer to God" must have been inspired by the devotional elements involved in achieving the immaculate helmet hair that was worn well into the 1960s. In fact, Priscilla Presley may be guilty of the most heinous of hair infractions worn on her wedding day. So prevalent was the use of hairsprays containing ozone-depleting propellants that in the mid 1970s the government issued a ban against the worst offenders—fluorocarbons.

In the late 1960s Vidal Sassoon created revolutionary angular and asymmetrical haircuts that went with the mod fashions of the times. Sassoon's styles were best worn on dark, shiny hair as embodied by Nancy Kwan or Penelope Tree. Finally, women were liberated from the tyranny of the blonde bombshell. But then just a few years later Farrah Fawcett's blonde winged hair created a stir, while beach blondes like Cheryl Tiegs and Christie Brinkley revived the "blondes have more fun" ethos. No doubt the big hair of the 1980s was a rebellion against the swinging hair of the 1960s.

Diana Ross may have understated the obvious when she said, "Hair has always been important." But more even than women, men have strong ties to their tresses—or lack thereof. Sampson lost his power when the vixenish Delilah snipped *his* manly mane, Bogey wore a rug, and Yul Brynner was known for his sexy bald pate. At age thirty, Ted Spiker, an editor at *Men's Health* and *Women's Health* magazines, shaved his full head of hair into a less-than-flattering horseshoe shape to see how his George Costanza 'do impacted his life. While women spend hours on hair, makeup, and fragrance, men are fairly limited to rearranging their hair and pruning their facial shrubbery. Do they feel the intense pressure to conform to the ideals of advertising geared toward men? Spiker said, "I know that I'm never going to look like an ad in a magazine, but I don't mind trying to get there. Do I feel bad about it? Sometimes."

As for dealing with bad hair days? Follow the favored distraction method of bombshells both past and present: break out the cleavage. They'll never notice your wilted bangs or split ends.

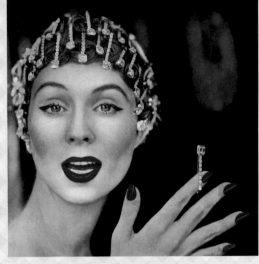

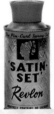
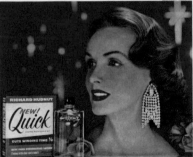
*J*n Greek mythology, Medusa began her life as a beautiful young maiden with silky hair. Medusa incurred the wrath of the goddess Athena who turned her into a snake-haired monster. Talk about a bad hair day.

*G*ently rub a dryer softening sheet over your static-y or hat hair to reduce that Marge Simpson effect.

Helena Rubinstein

Wash your hair with color!

5 Color-Tone Shampoos add natural color—without permanent dyes

HELENA RUBINSTEIN'S exciting new COLOR-TONE SHAMPOOS bring out the natural, bright, young tones your hair was meant to have.

You take no chances as with drastic dyes. The certified temporary color in COLOR-TONE SHAMPOO gives glamorous highlights, sparkling color—without any artificial look! In just one step, these amazing shampoos give you thorough cleansing, conditioning and naturalness!

Millions of women get the lively hair color they love with new COLOR-TONE SHAMPOO. You try it too.

Blonde-Tone makes a blonde more so, adds gold to light brown hair. *Red-Tone* plays up the flame, gives brown hair a chestnut look. *Brunette-Tone* gives dark hair dazzling warm depths. *Silver-Tone* adds shimmer to gray, white, ash blonde hair, corrects yellowing. *Brown-Glow* brings out red-gold lights in brown hair.

At leading department and drug stores.
Helena Rubinstein, 655 Fifth Avenue, New York 22, New York.

3-month supply ... 1.25
Giant size, 2.50

In 1937, Roma Whitney became one of the original Breck Girls. The 17 year old's image was registered as the company's trademark in 1951. A large collection of Breck Girl advertisements were featured in the January 2000 *Smithsonian Magazine*.

New bouncing Breck!

For bouncing hair

The only shampoo with Sartron to put new bounce into your hair.

New Breck Concentrate Shampoo bursts into delicious lather instantly. It rinses quickly, thoroughly. Leaves hair not just clean, but bouncing clean. It's got Sartron—a natural conditioner—a born manager—a real bouncer. Sartron helps hair stay lively lovely. Easier to curl, hold a curl longer. Try new bouncing Breck—in the bouncing tube. Two formulas: All-Family and For Dry Hair.

Beautiful Hair
BRECK

N E W

Beautiful Hair
Breck
Hair Set Mist

CONTAINS LIQUID LANOLIN
NET WEIGHT 4½ OZ

COPYRIGHT 1953 BY
JOHN H BRECK INC
Manufacturing Chemists
SPRINGFIELD · MASS · USA
PRINTED IN USA

Breck Hair Set Mist

A GENTLE, FRAGRANT SPRAY THAT HOLDS HAIR SOFTLY, BEAUTIFULLY IN PLACE FOR HOURS

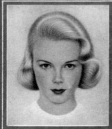

Breck Hair Set Mist is a fragrant spray, gentle as nature's mist, yet its delicate touch holds your hair softly in place for hours. After combing, a few brief sprays keep the hair beautifully in place.

When it's time for freshening, a damp comb renews your waves – no respraying is necessary.

Breck Hair Set Mist provides a quick and easy way to make lasting pin curls, too.

Fragrant as a bouquet, Breck Hair Set Mist contains lanolin, which leaves the hair soft to the touch and brings out the natural lustre and beauty of your hair.

Beautiful Hair

B R E C K

Available at Beauty Shops, Drug Stores, Department Stores and wherever cosmetics are sold. 4½ oz. $1.25; 11 oz. $2.00. Plus tax.

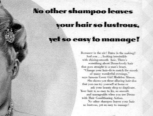

No other shampoo leaves your hair so lustrous, yet so easy to manage!

Romance in the air? Dance in the making! And you . . . looking irresistible with shining-smooth hair. There's something about Drene-lovely hair that goes straight to a man's heart. "Change your hair-do to match the mood of many wonderful evenings," says famous Cover Girl Madeline Mason. She shows you those alluring hair-dos that you can try yourself at home or ask your beauty shop to duplicate. Your hair is so easy to fix, so smooth and manageable when you use Drene with Hair Conditioning Action. No other shampoo leaves your hair so lustrous, yet so easy to manage!

IF SHE'S A SOPHISTICATE and loves you to look glamorous, try this bell-fluid upsweep. "Luvз Drene," says Madeline, "because it leaves my hair far more lustrous than any soap." Actually as much as 33% more luster! Since Drene is just a 2-1/2p shampoo, it never leaves any dulling film to hide so all soaps do.

IF SHE PREFERS SPORTS like bowling, she'll admire a tailored hair-do like this shiny shining braid. "I like to wear a scarf for active games," says Madeline, "but still show plenty of hair." Of course you'll want to show your hair too, when it's so lovely, full the natural brilliance is revealed by Drene with your first shampoo!

IF YOU'RE THE DEMURE TYPE who enjoys crowds? Then your hair must be near as lovely for close inspection. No unsightly dandruff to spoil your smooth groomed look . . . not when you're a Drene Girl! For this simple, graceful hair-do criss-cross your hair in back and hold with jewelled clips.

Drene

Shampoo with Hair Conditioning Action

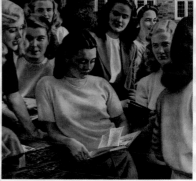

wherever women gather . . . **Just count those shining Lustre-Creme heads!**

Today, you see so many, many heads of glorious, beautiful hair in every town of all girls or women. These shining Lustre-Creme heads have all come about since the introduction of Lustre-Creme Shampoo, that remarkable "touch of magic" created by Kay Daumit for true hair loveliness. More and more women find that Lustre-Creme Shampoo leaves their hair with silken softness and natural, gleaming highlights. Not a soap, not a liquid, Lustre-Creme Shampoo is an amazing new dainty cream, that lathers luxuriously in hard or soft water—quickly (no special rinse)—vitally—inexpensively (many shampoos in the standard jar). Lustre-Creme Shampoo contains pure, gentle lanolin combined with secret ingredients, assures marvelous softness and obedience to the hair. Make your next shampoo a Lustre-Creme treatment and see how clean, fragrant, delightful your own hair can be. You will find Lustre-Creme Shampoo in attractive blue jars. At all cosmetic counters.

AT LAST! **A LIQUID SHAMPOO** THAT'S **EXTRA RICH !**

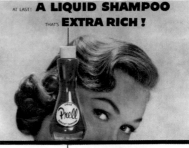

IT'S LIQUID **PRELL** for *Radiantly Alive Hair*

JUST POUR IT . . . and you'll see the glorious difference!

Exciting surprise for you—magical new Liquid Prell! It's extra rich— that's why Liquid Prell leaves your hair looking 'Radiantly Alive!' And how you'll love its unique, extra-rich formula. Bursts instantly into richer, more effective lather—rinses in a twinkle—leaving your hair easier to set. Shouldn't you try Extra-Rich Liquid Prell today? There's radiant beauty in every drop!

And you'll love PRELL CONCENTRATE— leaves hair extra clean . . . extra radiant!

Not a cream, not a liquid—Prell is that shampoo concentrate that cleans away cleansing ingredients, rinse far cleaner than any other shampoo! That's why Prell Concentrate leaves your hair extra clean, extra radiant!

PRELL

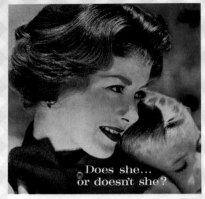

Does she...
or doesn't she?

Hair color so natural only her hairdresser knows for sure!

MISS CLAIROL® HAIR COLOR BATH

Henna, which provided Lucille Ball with her fiery red locks, has its roots in ancient Eastern and Islamic cultures, where intricate henna body painting began as a wedding ritual (and it is still practiced today).

New Beauty Miracle for Younger-Looking Hair!

NEW *Prell* leaves hair 'Radiantly Alive'

...actually more radiant than cream or soap shampoos!

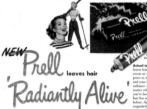

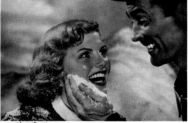

New Prell — for hair that's 'Radiantly Alive'... softer, smoother, younger looking!

Hair with the fresh young HALO look

is softer, brighter

Whistle Clean

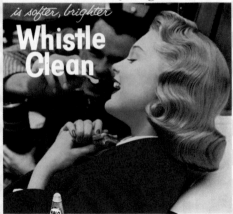

HALO SHAMPOO

—for clear, liquid Halo...unlike most shampoos...contains no greasy oils or soap. Nothing to interfere with cleaning action or dull your hair with heavy, dirt-catching film. Mild, gentle Halo leaves hair softer, brighter...whistle clean!

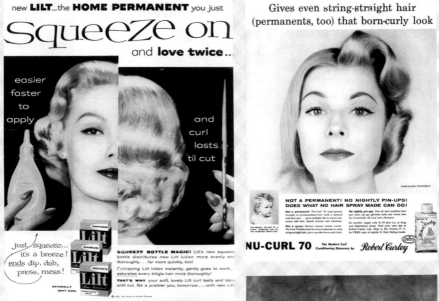

The active ingredient in
Pantene shampoo, panthenol,
is a vitamin derivative that was
discovered by Swiss medical
researchers during World War II.
They were searching for treatments
to help severe burn victims when
they made their discovery.

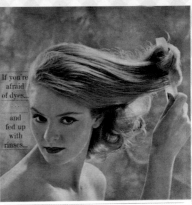

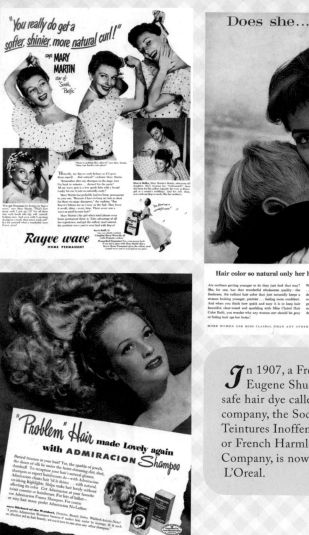

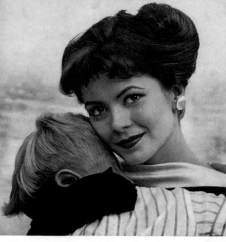

Does she...or doesn't she?

Hair color so natural only her hairdresser knows for sure!

Are mothers getting younger or do they just look that way? She, for one, has that wonderful wholesome quality—the freshness, the radiant hair color that just naturally keeps a woman looking younger, prettier ... feeling more confident. And when you think how quick and easy it is to keep hair beautiful, clear-toned and sparkling with Miss Clairol Hair Color Bath, you wonder why any woman ever should let gray or fading hair age her looks!

With Miss Clairol, finished color is always soft and ladylike ... lovely, natural-looking in any light. That's why hairdressers all over the world recommend Miss Clairol, use it every time to add young color to fading hair ... and to hide gray! *It takes only minutes, so silky and to look younger, more attractive!* Try Miss Clairol yourself. Today. In wonderful new Creme Formula or Regular.

MISS CLAIROL HAIR COLOR BATH

MORE WOMEN USE MISS CLAIROL THAN ANY OTHER HAIR COLORING

*I*n 1907, a French chemist named Eugene Shueller developed a safe hair dye called Aureole. His company, the Societe Francaise de Teintures Inoffensive pour Cheveux, or French Harmless Hair Coloring Company, is now better known as L'Oreal.

Which Twin has the Toni?

(see answer below)

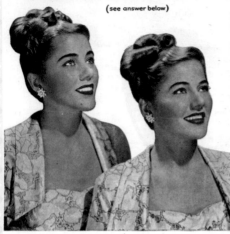

One Permanent Cost $15...the TONI only $2

Such deep luxurious waves. So soft, so natural-looking. You'll say your Toni Home Permanent is every bit as lovely as an expensive salon wave. But before trying Toni, you'll want the answers to these questions:

Will TONI work on my hair?
Yes, Toni waves any kind of hair that will take a permanent, including gray, dyed, bleached or baby fine hair.

Can I do it myself?
Sure. Every day thousands of women give themselves Toni Home Permanents. It's easy as rolling your hair up on curlers.

Will TONI save me time?
Definitely. The actual waving time is only 2 to 3 hours. And during that time you are free to do whatever you like.

How long will my TONI wave last?
Your Toni wave is guaranteed to last just as long as a $15 beauty shop permanent — or your money back.

Tune in "Give and Take"
2 p. m., EST, Saturday, CBS Network.

How much will I save with TONI?
The Toni Home Permanent Deluxe Kit with re-usable plastic curlers costs only $2 . . . Regular Kit with handy fiber curlers only $1.25. The Toni Refill Kit complete except for curlers is just $1. (Prices slightly higher in Canada).

Which twin has the TONI?
Lovely Jewel Bubnick of Miami Beach, says, "My sister, Ann, had an expensive beauty shop wave. I gave myself a Toni permanent —at home. And even our dates couldn't tell our permanents apart." Jewel, the twin with the Toni, is on the left.

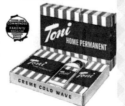

Toni
HOME PERMANENT

CREME COLD WAVE

Hair with the fresh young HALO look is softer, brighter

Whistle Clean

—for no other shampoo offers Halo's unique cleansing ingredient, so effective yet so mild. And there are no *unnecessary* ingredients in Halo. No greasy oils or creamy substances to interfere with cleaning action, no soap to leave dirt-catching film. Halo, even in *hardest* water, leaves hair softer, brighter, *whistle clean.*

HALO
SHAMPOO

91

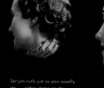
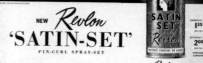
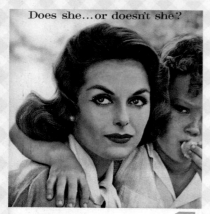
*I*t took a total of about eleven years to develop Head & Shoulders shampoo. In 1950 Procter & Gamble decided to create a dandruff shampoo. By the mid 1950s they discovered Pyrithione zinc, an ingredient to combat dandruff. The product was tested for another five years and was then known by a top-secret code name until its launch in fall 1961.

Don't burn the beauty
out of your hair
with drying
alcohol sprays

Every other leading spray-set sprays your hair with 80% to 95% alcohol. And alcohol can dry, dull, deaden hair . . . soon burn its beauty away.

New! The only spray-set with <u>no alcohol</u>
–builds beauty as it curls!

Such silky, soft curls! Never dry-looking.
Such shiny, springy curls! Never stiff, sticky or flaky.

Real dream stuff, this fabulous new Beauty Curl. Sets beauty . . . holds beauty . . . *builds* beauty! And without a drop of drying, burning alcohol that can rob your hair of the natural oils that protect its precious lustre.

No sticky lacquer or gummy fixative, either. Yet you can use it to set and to *hold!* And every time you spray it on, you can *see* an added glow. That's because Beauty Curl builds beauty from within. No wonder you get those soft, shiny curls that keep their joyous bounce even on the dampest day. Better get new Beauty Curl today!

A NEW *Richard Hudnut* DISCOVERY

Beauty Curl SPRAYS IN BEAUTY . . . SETS AND HOLDS NATURAL-LOOKING CURLS.

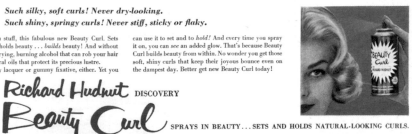

© 1957 Lambert-Hudnut Div.

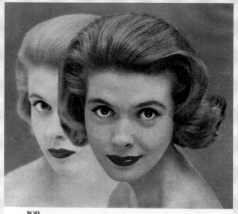

with ROUX...haircolor that looks as though it had always been your own!

The great gift of sparkling natural looking haircolor is that it helps you look – and feel – so much younger. And no matter what your coloring purpose may be, that's a gift Roux can bring you!

You may want to color gray hair, or simply to put a shining glow in hair that looks faded and dull. You may want to try a completely new haircolor, or to match your natural color. You may want a lasting hair-color, or a temporary one...or no color at all, but a lustrous hair lightening.

Whatever your desire, you'll find your answer in Roux, America's first family of haircolorings. For there's a Roux product designed for your specific purpose, and it imparts the natural look that is the mark of good taste. That is why hairstylists, whose livelihood depends on beauty, use more Roux haircolorings than any other?

So if your hairdresser doesn't do all it can and should for you, turn with confidence to Roux. Remember that "Roux means lovelier haircolor"...sparkling, natural looking haircolor and softer, more manageable hair condition!

ask your hairdresser why she prefers **ROUX**

Hair with the fresh young HALO look is softer, brighter
Whistle Clean

—for no other shampoo offers Halo's unique cleansing ingredient, so effective yet so mild. And there are no *unnecessary* ingredients in Halo. No greasy oils or creamy substances to interfere with cleaning action, no soap to leave dirt-catching film. Halo, even in *hardest* water, leaves hair softer, brighter, *whistle clean.*

HALO
SHAMPOO

𝒯 urbans, those weirdly glamorous head toppers popularized by femme fatales of the 1940s, were actually designed to cover up greasy hair. Shampoo was scarce during wartime and women refused to be seen in public with unwashed hair.

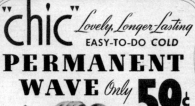

"chic"
Lovely, Longer-Lasting
EASY-TO-DO COLD
PERMANENT WAVE *Only* 59¢

COMPLETE
Including 50 Curlers

CERTIFIED
GUARANTEED

So Wonderful So Thrifty!

The "CHIC" home kit for only 59c contains everything needed for a truly lovely cold permanent wave including 50 curlers and a newly illustrated easy-to-follow direction booklet. "CHIC" is on sale at Hair Goods and Toiletry Counters everywhere.

Simple as A·B·C ... It's easy to give yourself a beautiful cold permanent wave right in the comforts of your own home. And, you'll be thrilled with the soft, exquisitely molded, natural looking curls and waves you get with a "CHIC" PERMANENT WAVE HOME KIT. "CHIC" requires no heat, no machines or dryers, no harmful chemicals or ammonia. Beauty-wise women and girls prefer "CHIC."

For all types of hair ..... Proven tests show that women using "CHIC" get the finest results possible. A "CHIC" permanent "takes" beautifully on every type of hair ... fine, medium or coarse ... bleached or dyed. Excellent for children's hair, too.

It's fun to style your own hair ... It's thrilling to be admired! Keep your hair looking lovely for every occasion. For "permanent" hair-beauty, use "CHIC."

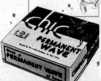

GET "chic" AT...DRUG STORES · DEPARTMENT STORES · VARIETY STORES · 5 AND 10c STORES

NEW!

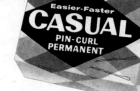

Easier-Faster
CASUAL
PIN-CURL PERMANENT

EASIEST
Pin-curl permanent...ever!

SET IT!

Set your pin-curls just as you always do. No need for anyone's help!

WET IT!

Apply CASUAL just once. 15 minutes later, rinse with clear water.

FORGET IT!

That's all there is to it! CASUAL is self-neutralizing. There's no resetting. Your work is finished.

Naturally lovely carefree curls that last for weeks!

With CASUAL your hair will be soft, naturally curly ... with all the body, the carefree beauty of curls just as you want them—perfect for the new softer natural look. Tonight—try CASUAL!

takes just 15 minutes more than setting your hair!
$1.50 PLUS TAX

95

JUST *One* *Shampoo*

... and your hair grows lovelier

CONTI'S olive oil castile safeguards the NATURAL OIL BALANCE of your hair

Your first shampoo proves it. Conti Castile Shampoo is scientifically good for your hair. End detergent dryness with its natural oil conditioning. Made with imported olive oil, Conti recaptures the bright natural luster ... the caressing softness. Your hair takes and holds waves beautifully, without damage to hair coloring. Why have dry, wispy, hard-to-manage hair? Conti Castile Shampoo will make it lovelier. Regular size, 57¢

USED BY LEADING HAIRDRESSERS

"Conti is our regular salon shampoo," says famous *Emile—Rockefeller Center.* "It is a favorite with leading hair stylists everywhere."

CONTI
CASTILE SHAMPOO
made with olive oil

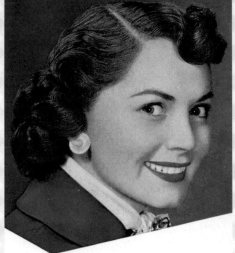

Dream girl, dream girl, beautiful Lustre-Creme Girl

Hair that gleams and glistens from a Lustre-Creme shampoo

Tonight!...Show him how much lovelier your hair can look...after a

Lustre-Creme Shampoo

Exclusive! This magical secret-blend lather with LANOLIN!
Exciting! This new three-way hair loveliness ...

1 **Leaves hair silken soft,** instantly manageable ... first wondrous result of a Lustre-Creme shampoo. Makes lavish, lanolin-blessed lather even in hardest water. No more unruly, soap-dulled locks. Leaves hair soft, obedient, for any style hair-do.

2 **Leaves hair sparkling** with star-bright sheen. No other shampoo has the same magic blend of secret ingredients plus gentle lanolin to bring out every highlight. No special rinse needed with Lustre-Creme Shampoo.

3 **Leaves hair fragrantly clean,** free of loose dandruff. Famous hairdressers insist on Lustre-Creme, the world's leading cream shampoo. Yes, tonight, show *him* a lovelier you—after a Lustre-Creme shampoo!

Not a soap! Not a liquid! But Kay Daumit's *cream* shampoo with lanolin. Jars: $2, $1. Jars and tubes: 49¢, 25¢.

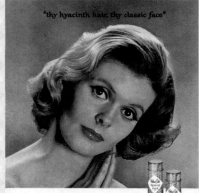

"thy hyacinth hair, thy classic face"

Your hair remembers its loveliest lines ... when it's

trained with Helene Curtis Spray Net®

If your hair tangles to pieces, is the fault perhaps your own? Are you using a mere pinsetting spray? Or are you brushing your hair while Helene Curtis intact isn't and its exclusive "control" ingredient? The secret isn't to set after but long-lasting pincurls. The it is always to hold your hair in place. Gradually, teasingly your curls get the habit of curling. These lovely waves remember their place from shampoo to shampoo. Use spray net faithfully, confident that even your hair will be linked to softest perfection—poetic perfection!

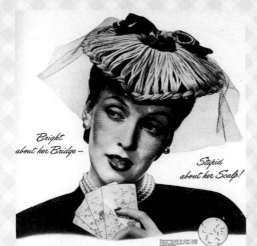

Bright about her Bridge —

Stupid about her Scalp!

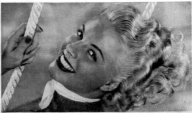
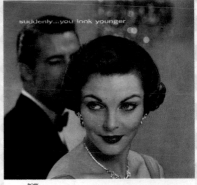

suddenly...you look younger

with ROUX...haircolor that looks as though it had always been your own!

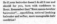

> *N*oted diva Marlene Dietrich once insisted that Max Factor sprinkle half an ounce of genuine gold dust into her wigs.

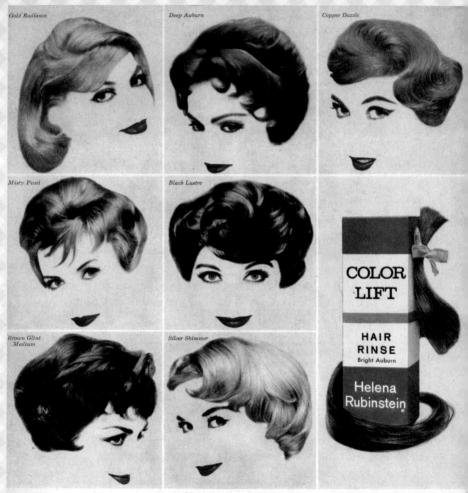

Gold Radiance

Deep Auburn

Copper Dazzle

Misty Pearl

Black Lustre

Brown Glint Medium

Silver Shimmer

COLOR
LIFT

HAIR
RINSE
Bright Auburn

Helena
Rubinstein

Choose your shade! One rinse keeps your hair glowing with color for weeks!

Only Helena Rubinstein could create COLOR LIFT
-the first color rinse that <u>lasts</u> <u>through</u> <u>5 shampoos</u>!

WISP STICK grooms unruly hair
at a stroke!

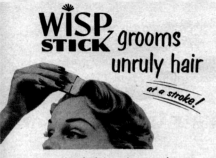

IT'S NEW! Now, for hair repair ... anywhere ... you'll carry a WISP-Stick*

Watch hair behave the WISP-Stick way! Just stroke it on, then comb hair. What a difference! Hair stays put, gleams with smoothness. No greasy, "plastered down" look with this amazing new hair cosmetic.

As handy as your lipstick in a smart little portable case. It's smooth going for the girl who carries a WISP-Stick!

- keeps stray wisps in place
- controls short ends
- tames wiry permanents
- keeps hair-do neat, manageable

Fits bag or make-up kit

$1 plus tax

at cosmetic counters
Slightly higher in Canada

Guaranteed by Good Housekeeping

...et, applied for
Good Grooming Products, Detroit, Mich.

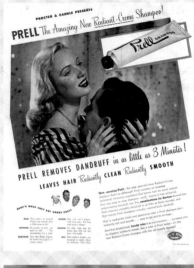

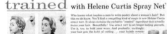
---

*S*noods were considered an elegant way to keep unruly hair under control while leaving the hairline showing. Sheer snoods were worn during the day, while elaborately crocheted snoods trimmed with ribbon or flowers were considered more appropriate for evening wear.

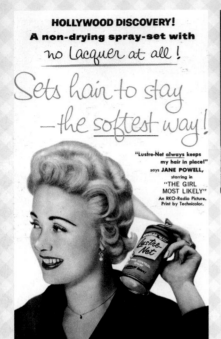

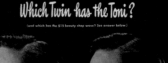

The first hairdryer was actually a modified vacuum cleaner.

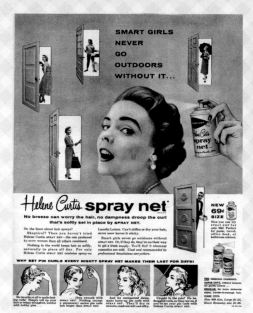
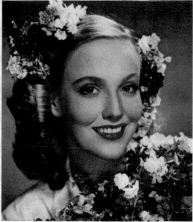
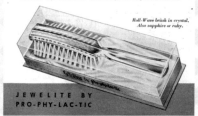
*T*he late 1960s saw a rise in the
popularity of natural hairstyles
with women growing their hair and
wearing it straight to the waist or
ornamented with flowers.

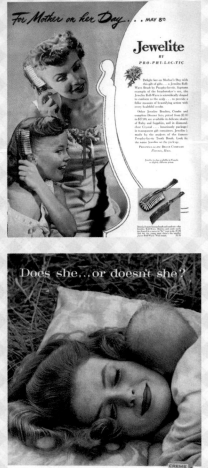
Wigs, popular in the 1950s, have been around for centuries. Catherine II of Russia, enraged at the prospect of a bad hair day, kept her wigmaker in an iron cage in her bedroom for over three years.

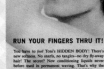

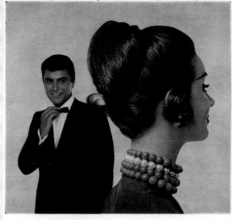

*I*n 1963 the popularity of the pillbox hat was resurrected. Images of First Lady Jackie Kennedy wearing her pink pillbox hat while cradling the president's head in her lap sparked the craze.

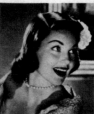
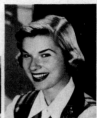
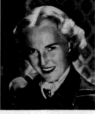
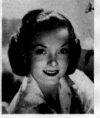

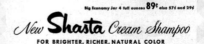

They put that $100 gleam in their hair with

Lady Wildroot Shampoo

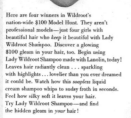

Janie King of E. St. Louis, Ill., says, "Lady Wildroot Shampoo gets my scalp pink-clean . . . washes away dirt and grime in a twinkling . . . gleams my hair without a special rinse."

Here are four winners in Wildroot's nation-wide $100 Model Hunt. They aren't professional models—just four girls with beautiful hair who *keep* it beautiful with Lady Wildroot Shampoo. Discover a glowing $100 gleam in your hair, too. Begin using Lady Wildroot Shampoo made with Lanolin, today! Leaves hair radiantly clean . . . sparkling with highlights . . . lovelier than you ever dreamed it could be. Watch how this *soapless* liquid cream shampoo whips to sudsy froth in seconds. Feel how silky soft it leaves your hair. Try Lady Wildroot Shampoo—and find the hidden gleam in *your* hair!

Lorraine Samson, New Brunswick, Can., says, "Lady Wildroot Shampoo gets my hair whistle-clean . . . leaves it with sunny highlights."

Lorna Kelly, East Orange, N.J., says, "Lady Wildroot Shampoo is so quick-sudsing - my hair gets cleaner sooner, stays cleaner longer."

Elizabeth Jane Lewis of Denver, Col., says, "Lady Wildroot Shampoo makes my hair so soft . . . it's fun to use the same grown-up shampoo Mommy does."

Lady Wildroot shampoo   gleams as it cleans— cleans as it gleams

You can win $100 too!

Send a snapshot or photo (not larger than 8 x 10 inches) showing your hair after using Lady Wildroot Shampoo, plus a Lady Wildroot Shampoo box top, to Lady Wildroot Shampoo Model Hunt, P. O. Box 189, New York 46, N. Y. Print your name and address on back of picture. If your photo is chosen, Wildroot will pay you $100 and your portrait may be painted by a famous artist and used in a Wildroot ad. Judges will be a New York artist and an art director, whose decisions are final. No photos returned. Offer good 60 days from the appearance of this magazine only. Send in your photo today.

Three Sizes 29¢ 59¢ 93¢

Lather hairdo shaped by Enrico Carusa

Drench your hair in luxury with Liquid Prell . . . *the extra-rich shampoo!*

*L*ucille Ball's poodle hairdo wasn't the only canine craze to surface in the 1950s. Girls became obsessed with full skirts with poodle appliqués. Other faves included patches of records, flowers, animals, and cars.

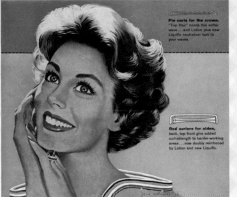
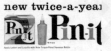
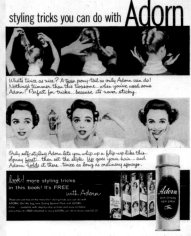

T he Civil Rights movement of the mid 1960s spawned the Afro, a hairstyle that reflected the aesthetic of "black is beautiful." Afros were considered a rebellion against the concept of straightening or over-processing African American hair to emulate the predominantly white culture.

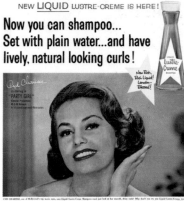

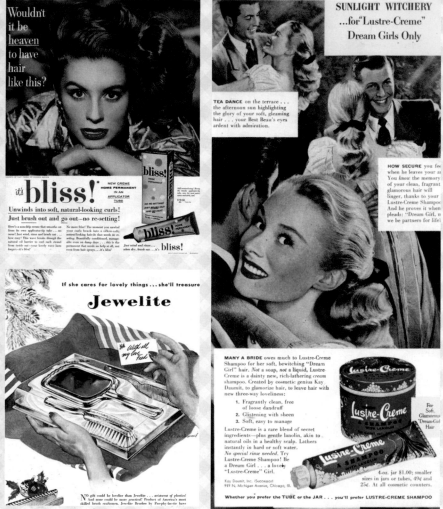

Wouldn't it be heaven to have hair like this?

it's bliss!

NEW CREME HOME PERMANENT IN AN APPLICATOR TUBE

Unwinds into soft, natural-looking curls!
Just brush out and go out—no re-setting!

Here's a non-drip creme that smooths on from its own applicator-tip tube ... so neat! Just wind, rinse and brush out ... how easy! This wave breaks through the natural oil barrier to curl each strand from inside out—your lovely wave lasts longer—it's bliss!

No more frizz! The moment you unwind your curls brush into a silken-soft, natural-looking hair-do that needs no re-setting. Beautifully conditioned, manageable even on damp days ... this is the permanent that needs no help at all, and even from hair sprays ... it's bliss!

Just wind and rinse ...
when dry, brush out ... it's bliss!

bliss!
HOME PERMANENT

If she cares for lovely things ... she'll treasure

Jewelite

With all my love Fred

NO gift could be lovelier than Jewelite ... aristocrat of plastics! And none could be more practical! Product of America's most skilled brush craftsmen, Jewelite Brushes by Pro-phy-lac-tic have

---

SUNLIGHT WITCHERY
...for "Lustre-Creme"
Dream Girls Only

TEA DANCE on the terrace ... the afternoon sun highlighting the glory of your soft, gleaming hair ... your Best Beau's eyes ardent with admiration.

HOW SECURE you feel when he leaves your arms. You know the memory of your clean, fragrant glamorous hair will linger, thanks to your Lustre-Creme Shampoo. And he proves it when he pleads: "Dream Girl, shall we be partners for life!"

MANY A BRIDE owes much to Lustre-Creme Shampoo for her soft, bewitching "Dream Girl" hair. Not a soap, not a liquid, Lustre-Creme is a dainty new, rich-lathering cream shampoo. Created by cosmetic genius Kay Daumit, to glamorize hair, to leave hair with new three-way loveliness:

1. Fragrantly clean, free of loose dandruff
2. Glistening with sheen
3. Soft, easy to manage

Lustre-Creme is a rare blend of secret ingredients—plus gentle lanolin, akin to natural oils in a healthy scalp. Lathers instantly in hard or soft water. No special rinse needed. Try Lustre-Creme Shampoo! Be a Dream Girl ... a lovely "Lustre-Creme" Girl.

Kay Daumit, Inc. (Successor)
919 N. Michigan Avenue, Chicago, Ill.

For Soft, Glamorous 'Dream-Girl' Hair

Lustre-Creme
WITH LANOLIN

Lustre-Creme
A SHAMPOO
WITH LANOLIN

4-oz. jar $1.00; smaller sizes in jars or tubes, 49¢ and 25¢. At all cosmetic counters.

Whether you prefer the TUBE or the JAR ... you'll prefer LUSTRE-CREME SHAMPOO

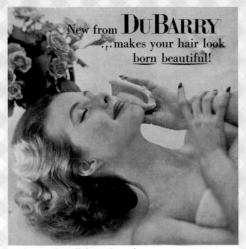
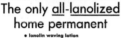
*a*verage humans have about 100,000 hairs on their head, and lose an average of 40 to 100 strands of hair a day. Blondes have more hair than dark-haired people. (Is that why blondes have more fun?)

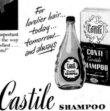

ALL *Smart* GIRLS SAY NO! NO! NO!

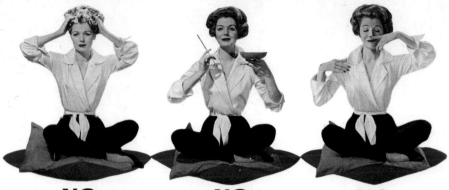

NO
shampooing!

NO
mixing!

NO
odor!

Totally New!

Fashion 'Quick'

The Salon-Tested Home Permanent

Shampoos each curl as it locks in your wave!

**FASHION 'QUICK' contains exclusive "Clean Curl" Neutralizer
...the amazing Built-in Shampoo!**

Imagine a permanent that even washes your hair for you!
Ends forever the 3 big home permanent problems. No shampooing–
before or after waving. No mixing, measuring, messing with
neutralizers. No "perm" odor. Leaves your hair fresh and clean...
sweet enough to kiss right after waving! For the most beautiful
wave you have ever had...in half the time...with half the work...
get Fashion 'Quick'. *Guaranteed* to take! *Guaranteed* to last!

Regular—for normal hair. Gentle—for bleached or damaged hair.
Super—for hard to wave hair (recommended for children)

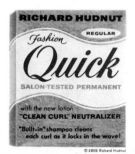

RICHARD HUDNUT

Fashion

Quick

SALON-TESTED PERMANENT

with the new lotion
"CLEAN CURL" NEUTRALIZER

"Built-in" shampoo cleans
each curl as it locks in the wave!

New *Fashion* 'Quick' Home Permanent
by **RICHARD HUDNUT**

© 1959 Richard Hudnut

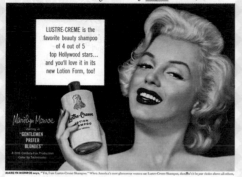

Thrilling Beauty News *for users of* <u>Liquid</u> **Shampoos!**

LUSTRE-CREME is the favorite beauty shampoo of 4 out of 5 top Hollywood stars... and you'll love it in its new Lotion Form, too!

Marilyn Monroe
starring in
"GENTLEMEN PREFER BLONDES"
A 20th Century-Fox Production
Color by Technicolor

MARILYN MONROE says, "Yes, I use Lustre-Creme Shampoo." When America's most glamorous women use Lustre-Creme Shampoo, shouldn't it be your choice above all others,

Now! Lustre-Creme Shampoo *also* in New Lotion Form!

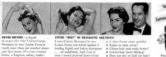

NEVER BEFORE—a liquid shampoo like this! Lustre-Creme Shampoo in new Lotion Form is much more than just another shampoo that pours. It's a one creamy lotion, a fragrant, satiny, easier-to-use lotion, that brings Lustre-Creme pleasure to your hair with every heavenly shampoo!

VOTED "BEST" IN DRAMATIC USE-TESTS!

Lustre-Creme Shampoo in new Lotion Form was voted against 4 leading liquid and lotion shampoos ... all unlabeled. And *3 out of every 5 women preferred Lustre-Creme* in new Lotion Form over each competing shampoo tested—for these important reasons:

• Lather forms more quickly!
• Easier to rinse away!
• Cleans hair and scalp better!
• Leaves hair more shining!
• Does not dry or dull the hair!
• Leaves hair tasting so fragrant!
• Hair has better fragrance!
• More economical to use!

Prove it to Yourself—
Lustre-Creme in new Lotion Form is the **best** liquid shampoo yet!

Yes! Now take your choice.

Famous **Cream** Form...or new Lotion Form

Famous Cream Form in jars or tubes, 27¢ to $1. (Big creamy size $1). New Lotion Form in handy bottle, 30¢ to $1.

POUR IT ON—OR CREAM IT ON! In famous Cream Form, Lustre-Creme is America's favorite cream shampoo. And all its beauty-bringing qualities are in the new Lotion Form. Whichever form you prefer, handle-filtered Lustre-Creme will leave your hair shining clean, eager to wave, never dull or dry.

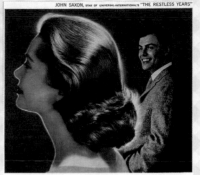

JOHN SAXON, STAR OF UNIVERSAL-INTERNATIONAL'S "THE RESTLESS YEARS"

"You can always tell a Halo girl...you can tell by the shine of her hair"

Give <u>your</u> hair that <u>extra shine</u>, too with today's Halo...

the modern shampoo with <u>extra-shining</u> action

♥ Halo shines as it cleans—with the purest, mildest cleansing ingredient possible!

♥ Halo leaves extra shine as it rinses—with the fastest, most thorough rinsing action ever!

With today's Halo it's so easy for your hair to have that extra shine. So satin-bright, satin-smooth, too—so manageable. Try it today in its modern beauty bottle.

*Halo glorifies as it cleans
...with extra shining action.*

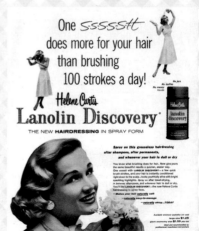

One Sssssttt does more for your hair than brushing 100 strokes a day!

Helene Curtis
Lanolin Discovery
THE NEW **HAIRDRESSING** IN SPRAY FORM

Spare what brushing does for hair. Now give yours the same beautiful results a quicker, easier way.
One ssssstt with LANOLIN DISCOVERY—a few quick brush strokes, and your hair is instantly conditioned right down to the scalp—looks youthfully alive with bright sparkling highlights. Spray on after towel-drying, in between shampoos, and whenever hair is dull or dry. You'll like **LANOLIN DISCOVERY**—the new Helene Curtis hairdressing in spray form.

—*Makes your hair naturally soft*
—*naturally easy-to-manage*
—*naturally shiny...TODAY*

Available economy (models size and large size $1.25 giant economy size $1.50 plus tax ideal and recommended by professional hairdressers everywhere)

---

a weekly celebrity news magazine, *Look*, was published from 1937 to 1971. It was heavy on photographs of glamorous hairstyles and celebrity beauty tricks and was considered a glossier version of *Life* magazine.

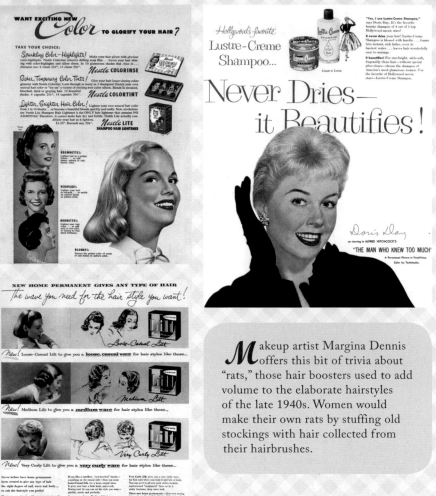

Makeup artist Margina Dennis offers this bit of trivia about "rats," those hair boosters used to add volume to the elaborate hairstyles of the late 1940s. Women would make their own rats by stuffing old stockings with hair collected from their hairbrushes.

Lovely hair deserves fine care

buy a better comb
...a DUPONT comb!

so strong!   *so smooth!*   *so beautiful!*

Need a strong comb? Want a smooth comb? Like a pretty comb?
Then Du Pont's for you!★ Du Pont Combs have strong, firm teeth. The
smooth, smooth plastic won't split your hair or scratch your
scalp. And the colors are bright, sparkling, go with everything!★ Today
one out of four people uses Du Pont Combs. There's a reason. Next time you
buy a comb, look for the Du Pont oval. Prices: 10¢, 15¢, 25¢, 50¢
at drug, department or 10¢ stores.

Better buy **Du Pont Combs**

BETTER THINGS FOR BETTER LIVING . . . *THROUGH CHEMISTRY*

111

Chapter 4
The Scent of Beauty

❖❖❖◆❖ ▣ ❖◆❖❖❖

According to a recent poll in the *New York Post*, Elizabeth Taylor is considered the most beautiful movie actress of all time, followed closely by Ava Gardner, Grace Kelly, Sophia Loren, Marilyn Monroe, and Audrey Hepburn. These top six glamour goddesses were all genetically gifted, but they also seemed to waft the scent of sensuality and classic feminine beauty. In the era of the "Sweet Smell of Success," not only was publicity manufactured, but so were the increasingly available mass-marketed accoutrements of attraction. Many women wore store-bought signature fragrances, which were frequently heady (and heavy) mixtures of floral, musk, and Oriental scents that were popular at the time.

Rochelle Bloom, president of the Fragrance Foundation, admits that she does not have one signature scent, but rather prefers to experiment with new favorites that match her wardrobe and her mood. When asked about the main differences between fragrance in the past as opposed to now, Bloom says that in the past "women wore fragrance to please a man, or to please and attract someone else. Today they wear it for themselves." She also considers fragrance choice to be an extension of self—your personality and identity.

Of all the cosmetic advertising of the mid-century, ads for perfume seemed to be the farthest removed from reality. Taking the concept of a living doll to extremes, some ads displayed a faintly morose looking doll in a variety of wardrobes and poses. The chatty ad copy ensured that by using their fragrance, you'd look both fresh and feminine.

Dainty seemed to be an adjective of choice in advertising of that era, and considering that the average shoe size in the 1950s was said to be about a 5 1/2 while in our own times it's an 8 (though celebutante Paris Hilton, she of the petite pooch and minute waist, is said to wear a size 11 shoe), they might actually have been on to something. Perfumes promised to keep you "fragrantly dainty" with a "liquid skin sachet." Not only that, you could "bathe your way to beauty." One spritz could bestow upon you a "fresh, young feeling" ensuring that you were nothing short of being a "hostess to loveliness." A mere shake of body powder left you not only cool, but also smooth and, of course, dainty.

If looking and smelling great was the ideal, sweating and smelling bad was a fate to be avoided at all costs—and through liberal use of costly beauty products. One shudders at the thought of the repercussions of body odor on a proper young lady's social standing. New Fresh stick deodorant was the "modern way to be safe!" Mum Mist promised to protect "even the two in five who perspire freely." And Colgate's VETO allowed you to "Say No, No to underarm 'O."

Was the advertising industry of the time guilty of feeding off of women's insecurities by exhorting these miracle products? Lester Barnett, a recent inductee into the Medical Advertising Hall of Fame, begs to differ. In his opinion "Advertising works powerfully as a supporter and enhancer of aspirations rather than as a feeder on insecurities. Look deeper than the benefit of not smelling bad to the bigger benefits that a woman herself seeks." He suggests that we try not to blame advertising for what society (including women) wants women to be. And in those times women wanted to be polished, odorless, and dainty.

During the swinging 1960s, dainty gave way to twiggy, literally, as the gently rounded models with hourglass figures of the 1940s and 1950s were replaced by bonnie, bony lovelies from across the pond. Jean Shrimpton, Jane Birkin, Penelope Tree, and Twiggy Lawson embodied the latest beauty ideals with their coltish figures, endless legs, and doe-like eyes.

Dainty, twiggy, or otherwise, beauty is all about being comfortable in your own skin—however you may choose to scent it.

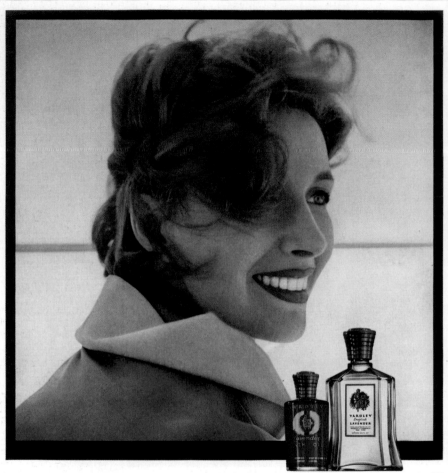

Lavender bath oil $1.75   Long-lasting Lavender essence from $1.10
(BOTH PLUS TAX)

Enjoy the fresh, young feeling
that Yardley Lavender gives you

No other fragrance can make you feel so fresh, so charming, all day long. Because Yardley Lavender is more than a delightful scent. It's a feeling... lighthearted, fresh and wonderful! And you know you look wonderful, when you *feel* wonderful. Choose Yardley Lavender in many forms; give it as proud gifts. Created in England, made in U.S.A. Yardley of London, Inc., 620 Fifth Avenue, N.Y.C.

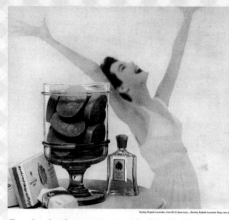

For the freshest, youngest feeling in the world

Here's a delightful way to feel fresh as a flower, light as air and young as laughter all day long. It's the lightning lift you get from Yardley English Lavender. Nothing in the world makes you feel so young, so fresh, so charming!

And it's so easy . . . a quick clean-up with Lavender soap, a fast splash-on of Lavender itself, can make you feel unbelievably refreshed and radiant in just a matter of minutes.

The soap's creamy, rich foam gently cleanses . . . leaves your skin soft complexion fresh and glowing. Famous and loved the world over, Yardley English Lavender Soap is fine-milled to last a long, long time . . . lathers freely down to the tiniest sliver. Made from a unique formula which is one of Yardley's most closely guarded secrets, it imparts the exhilarating fragrance . . . the stimulating feeling of English Lavender.

Throughout the day, make the cool, fresh lift of Lavender itself part of your loveliness. When you begin to feel weary, splash it on wrists, forehead and the hollow of your throat and revel in its refreshing, tingling fragrance.

Nothing in the world makes you feel so young, so fresh, so charming as Yardley English Lavender. Discover this for yourself by using Yardley English Lavender Soap and Yardley English Lavender Toilet Essence . . . enjoy its other fragrant forms, too. You'll find them all at your favorite drug or department store.

Obey Yardley, in all the world, brings you the fresh, young feeling of English Lavender. Blending the oil of English Lavender blossoms with precious ingredients from the earth's far corners, they achieve a fragrance that's truly unique.

Yardley products for America are created in England and finished in the U.S.A. from the original English formula, combining imported and domestic ingredients. Yardley of London, Inc., 620 Fifth Ave., N.Y.C.

Yardley *English* **Lavender**

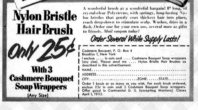

*D*esigner Gabrielle "Coco" Chanel called her first perfume "Chanel No. 5" because five was her lucky number. It became the world's best-selling perfume, and was said to be Marilyn Monroe's signature scent.

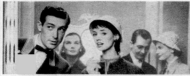

NEW MUM MIST PROTECTS EVEN THE 2 IN 5 WHO PERSPIRE FREELY

Here's deodorant protection you never thought possible!

New Mum Mist spray deodorant stops perspiration *instantly* and for hours. Contains miracle hexachlorophene to prevent odor *all day long*—even if you are one of the 2 in 5 who perspire freely.

No more messy running or dripping!

Mum Mist sprays on, stays on. It dries fast—won't run, won't drip. Completely safe for normal skin—doesn't damage delicate fabrics. For protection that's fast, protection that lasts— get new Mum Mist!

At all toiletries counters **59¢**

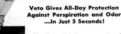

Say NO, NO to Underarm "O"
with Colgate's Super-Effective New VETO

Veto Gives All-Day Protection Against Perspiration and Odor —In Just 5 Seconds!

New Veto positively says no, no to underarm "O". Super-effective Veto stops odor instantly ... checks perspiration more effectively! It's an exclusive "wonder-formula."

Veto is light, fluffy—smooths on and absorbs as easily as vanishing cream. Never cakes or dries out in the jar. Has a delightful fragrance you'll love. And it's mild, won't irritate normal skin. Harmless to fabrics.

Guard daintiness from bath to bath. Use super-effective Veto daily. Get it now at any cosmetic counter.

Veto Protection Lasts from Bath to Bath!

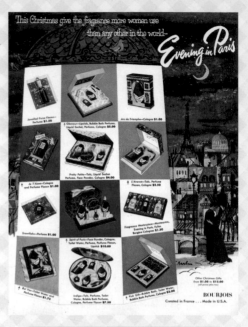

This Christmas give the fragrance more women use than any other in the world—

Evening in Paris

BOURJOIS
Created in France . . . Made in U.S.A.

*C*aron Paris created "Royal Bain de Champagne" perfume in the 1940s to cheer people up during the privation of war. The fragrance was meant to make the wearer feel pampered and as though they could "escape the world to a time of lavish Parisian parties."

116

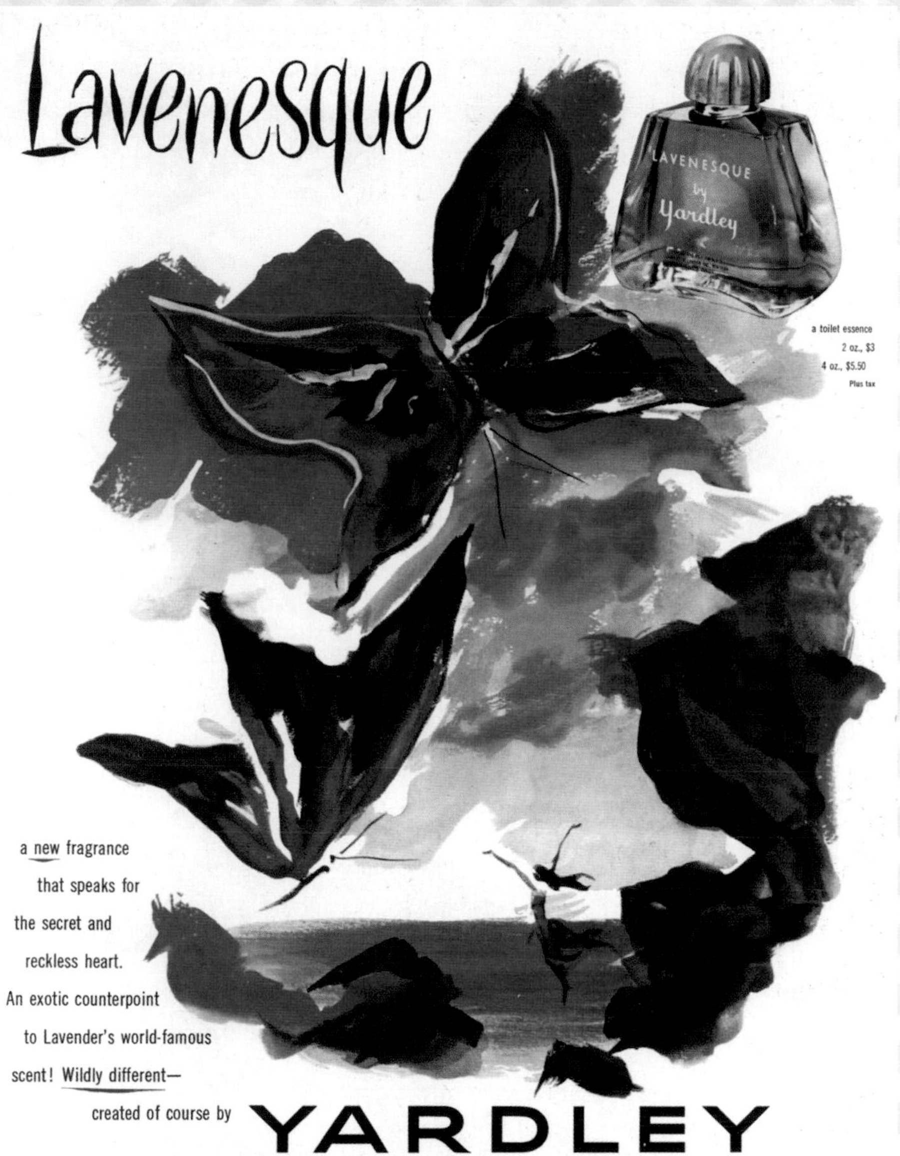

Lavenesque

LAVENESQUE
by
Yardley

a toilet essence
2 oz., $3
4 oz., $5.50
Plus tax

a new fragrance
that speaks for
the secret and
reckless heart.
An exotic counterpoint
to Lavender's world-famous
scent! Wildly different—
created of course by

YARDLEY

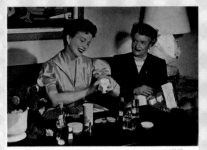

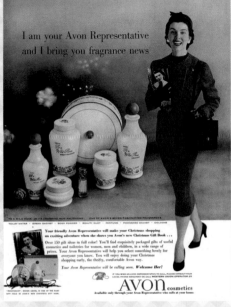

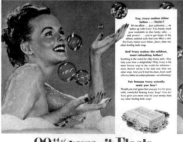

Christian Dior's perfume, "Poison," is a sexy and completely non-toxic scent, more about company image than actual danger. In the 1930s, the FDA produced shocking images of a beautiful woman blinded by Lash Lure, a lash-darkening agent.

BLESSED MOMENT...ALL YOUR OWN !

Shut the door on all the noise and bustle of the day . . . the children's chatter, the kitchen's clatter, your own thousand-and-one busy steps.

Run a warm full tub, slip off your clothes, step in and stretch out . . . *lazily* . . . letting the water ripple gently over all of you, throat to toes. Relax . . . and feel the long day's cares float clean away.

Make this moment all-your-own an extra-blessed one, with bland, caressing, gentle Palmolive. Smooth its quick, thick lather over face, throat, shoulders, all of you.

Your skin is cleansed swiftly, completely . . . and gently. For Palmolive is made with olive and palm oils—nature's finest beauty aids—*costliest oil* blend used for any leading soap. These vegetable oils (no animal fats)

are the only oils used in making Palmolive. And this is true of no other leading soap. Yet, for all its costliest oil blend, Palmolive costs *you* no more than the others. That is because Palmolive is the largest selling beauty soap in all the world.

So ask yourself, today, and answer truly . . . will anything less than Palmolive do for *your* all-over complexion?

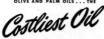

MAKE IT EXTRA-BLESSED...

Choose PALMOLIVE

MADE WITH OLIVE AND PALM OILS . . . THE

Costliest Oil

BLEND USED FOR ANY LEADING SOAP

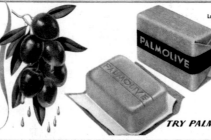

Look for the **NATURAL OLIVE COLOR**! It comes from olive and palm oils . . . nothing else!

IT'S NEW! MAN-SIZE, BATH-SIZE PALMOLIVE! Extra-big, longer-lasting for your tub and shower. The whole family cheers for it! Economical, too. Ask your dealer for Bath-Size Palmolive.

TRY PALMOLIVE...NOW !

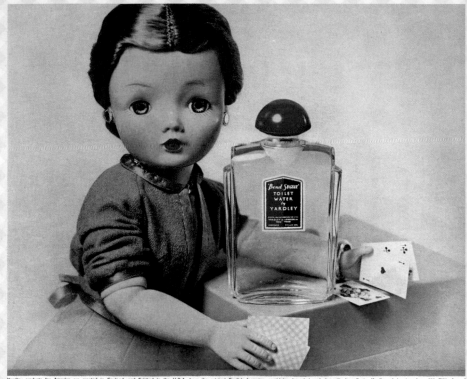

To make you feel especially feminine

YARDLEY fragrances ... of course

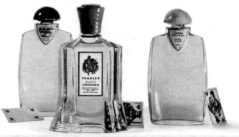

Which of these lovely, lingering scents is for you?
The vibrant sophistication of Bond Street?
Delicately exotic Lotus? Perhaps it's April Violets,
rain-sweet and incurably romantic. Or is your one
and only love the fresh, lighthearted gaiety of Lavender?
Not an easy choice to make—but a delightful one.
These toilet waters and colognes from $1.35 plus tax.

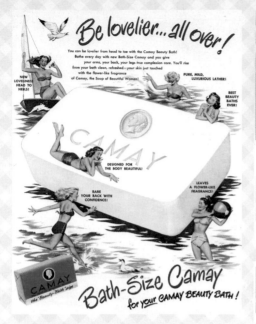
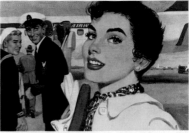

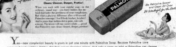
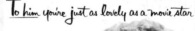
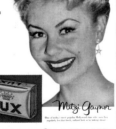
The average person can distinguish up to 10,000 different smells. As people age their sense of smell diminishes, so by the time you're sixty the perfume you wore at age twenty will smell completely different to you.

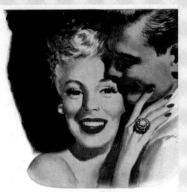

Try Palmolive's Famous "Beauty Lather" For Something

Thrillingly New!

New **Fragrance!**
New **Charm!**
New **Allure!**

And Doctors Prove You, Too, may win a Lovelier Complexion using nothing but Palmolive Soap!

Millions of women will prefer "Beauty Lather" Palmolive . . . the minute they try it! For Palmolive Soap's new flower-fresh fragrance means new allure, new charm.

And proper cleansing with Palmolive is so effective that *all types of skin*—young, old,

oily—respond to it quickly. Dull, drab skin looks brighter—coarse-looking skin finer!

So do as 36 doctors advised 1285 women, many with complexion problems. Wash your face with Palmolive Soap, massaging for one minute with Palmolive's wonderful "Beauty Lather." Rinse! Do this 3 times a day for 14 days. It's that simple.

Yes, doctors *proved* it could bring 2 out of 3 women lovelier complexions. Get Palmolive Soap and start today!

Use it in tub or shower. The alluring new fragrance of Palmolive's "Beauty Lather" leaves you even lovelier all over!

Get Bath Size Palmolive, too!

"ah-h! my Ivory Bath it's a pleasure... pure pleasure!"

Yes, there's more lather... faster lather... in an Ivory bath!

It's so relaxing to sink into an Ivory bath! You don't grope for soap—Ivory floats right into your hand. No wait for lather—that husky cake of Ivory fairly *bursts* into rich, foamy suds! For Ivory makes more lather, faster, than any other leading bath soap!

There's Ivory's famous mildness ... and such a clean, fresh odor!

It's pure delight—the gentle caress of silky Ivory suds. For Ivory Soap is 99 ⁴⁴⁄₁₀₀ % pure ... mild as mild. Why, more doctors advise Ivory for skin care than any other soap. And that clean, fresh-smelling Ivory lather leaves you so refreshed! All aglow and ready to go!

You get more for your money, too!

Yes, mild Ivory . . . pure Ivory . . . floating Ivory . . . actually costs you *less!* Gives you more soap for your money than any other leading bath soap!

99 ⁴⁴⁄₁₀₀ % pure...it Floats

"The whole family agrees on Ivory!"

America's Favorite Bath Soap!

While floral scents are the most popular fragrance, there isn't a perfumer alive who would create a fragrance from the Amorphophallus Titanium or "corpse flower." When the flower is in bloom, it emits a repulsive scent similar to a dead body.

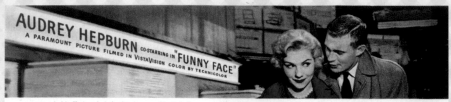

AUDREY HEPBURN A PARAMOUNT PICTURE FILMED IN VISTAVISION COLOR BY TECHNICOLOR CO-STARRING IN "FUNNY FACE"

SHE: Audrey Hepburn looks lovelier than ever, doesn't she?   **HE:** Yes, she does—and so do you!

To <u>him</u>

you're just as lovely

as a movie star

. . . he's *your* special audience . . . he loves to look *at you*. That's a wonderful thought! And here's another one. Daily Lux care can do as much to keep *your* skin fresh and glowing, as it does for Audrey Hepburn. Like 9 out of 10 Hollywood stars, lovely Audrey always uses Lux.

Cosmetic lather is the secret

New Lux lather has a beneficial *cosmetic* action on skin. It actually helps maintain the proper moisture balance so essential to a radiant complexion.

New Lux is sealed in Gold Foil

. . . to protect its *cosmetic* lather, dazzling whiteness, wonderful fragrance. You don't have to be a movie star to have a movie star's complexion—that's the beauty of new Lux in Gold Foil!

9 out of 10

Hollywood Stars

use —

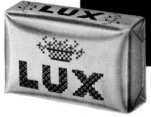

Audrey Hepburn

. . . dark hair, dark eyes, womanly grace and gamin charm . . . all part of lovely Audrey's appeal. Then there's her complexion—fresh, glowing—and cared for with new Lux!

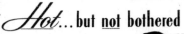

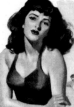

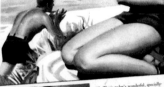

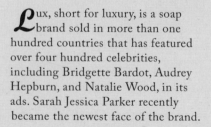

*L*ux, short for luxury, is a soap brand sold in more than one hundred countries that has featured over four hundred celebrities, including Bridgette Bardot, Audrey Hepburn, and Natalie Wood, in its ads. Sarah Jessica Parker recently became the newest face of the brand.

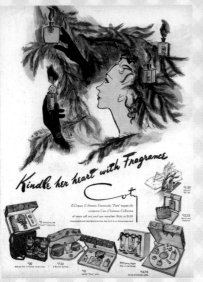

Kindle her heart with Fragrance

Coty

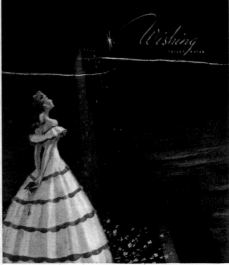

Wishing TOILET WATER

*G*ood perfume counters contain a bowl of coffee beans to help neutralize the effects of the heady scents that you've just inhaled, allowing you to process new ones.

Avon's enchanting new fragrance . . . spellbinding as the first star . . . romantic as a new moon! *Wishing* is everything your feminine heart could desire in a cooling, flower-fresh toilet water. The Avon Representative will bring *Wishing* Toilet Water direct to you in your home. Welcome her when she calls . . . be a hostess to loveliness.

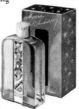

Wishing Toilet Water Commemorates Avon's 61st Anniversary—Service Through Friendly Calls since 1886.

Avon cosmetics

IN RADIO CITY, NEW YORK

126

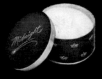

MIDNIGHT DUSTING POWDER $1

MIDNIGHT COLOGNE $1

MIDNIGHT BLUE ICE
STICK COLOGNE $1

MIDNIGHT LIPSTICK PERFUME COMBINATION $1

MIDNIGHT
by TUSSY

means romance...for you

A fragrance as exciting as a meeting by moonlight...that's Midnight! And a vivid pink lipstick color...with a touch of lilac...that's Midnight, too! Wear them both morning, noon and Midnight.   ALL PRICES PLUS TAX

Only one soap gives your skin this exciting Bouquet

The secret of dainty, romantic appeal is really amazingly simple!

Popular girls have known this secret for 80 years... so do as they do. Bathe every day with Cashmere Bouquet Soap, to surround yourself with a lingering, bewitching *fragrance men love!* A fragrance that comes only from a secret wedding of rare perfumes far more costly than you would expect to find in any soap.
Today, tomorrow, and *every day*... use exquisite Cashmere Bouquet Soap in your bath, and for your complexion, too!

Cashmere
Bouquet

Cashmere Bouquet

Adorns your skin with the fragrance men love—

NOW
IN
RED ROSES

NEW
AFTER BATH
FRESHENERS
BY
YARDLEY

YARDLEY
Red Roses
AFTER BATH
FRESHENER

English Lavender   April Violets

Prolong that delicious showered-with-red-roses feeling all day!
Splash on fragrant Yardley After Bath Freshener *lavishly.*
A delicate deodorant protects your freshness, emollients put
a silken "finishing touch" to your skin, prevent chapping.

*Enjoy After Bath Freshener in NEW Red Roses, unforgettable
true rose scent, English Lavender or April Violets, $1.85 plus tax.*

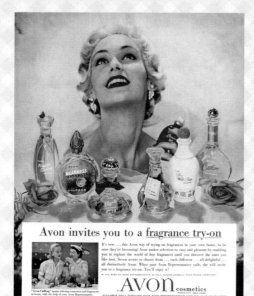

Avon invites you to a <u>fragrance try-on</u>

It's new . . . this Avon way of trying on fragrances in your own home, to be sure they're becoming! Avon makes selection so easy and pleasant by enabling you to explore the world of fine fragrances until you discover the ones you like best. Seven scents to choose from . . . each different . . . all delightful . . . all distinctively Avon. When your Avon Representative calls, she will invite you to a fragrance try-on. You'll enjoy it!

IF YOU WISH AN AVON REPRESENTATIVE TO CALL, PLEASE CONSULT YOUR PHONE DIRECTORY

"Avon Calling" means selecting cosmetics and fragrances at home, with the help of your Avon Representative.

AVON cosmetics

RADIO CITY NEW YORK

AVAILABLE ONLY THROUGH YOUR AVON REPRESENTATIVE WHO CALLS AT YOUR HOME

*S*kin-So-Soft body oil, one of Avon's top selling brands, is also popular as a bug repellent. Bugs can't seem to stay on oil slick skin and are repelled by the citronella scent.

blossom-fresh
as spring-garden lilacs

Wrisley *lilac-fragrance*
Bath Superbe Soap

Heavenly, flower-fresh Lilac fragrance skillfully blended into a luxurious, creamy-lathering, *rich* base. If you've never used Bath Superbe Soap, you don't know how wonderful soap can be! Smooth-textured—gentle and lotion-mild.

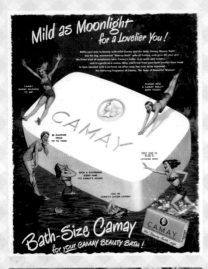
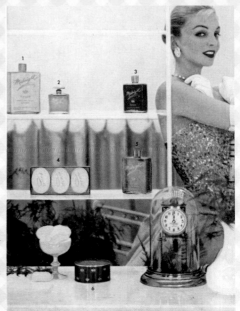
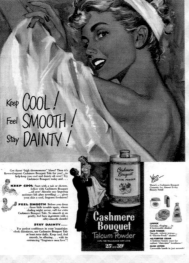

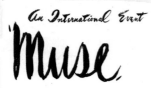

An International Event
'Muse,

A GREAT NEW PERFUME IS A RARE EVENT

*Mere fragrance does not make a perfume...
just as paint does not make a painting...
nor sounds a symphony.*

*'Muse' is the climax of eight years of sensitive composing...
marked by many moments of discouragement but crowned
by ultimate triumph... eight years of subtle, masterful
blending of more than thirty ingredients to create
a new masterpiece in perfumes. A new perfume
born in the heart of Paris, 'Muse' is destined to become
a classic growing ever greater with the passage of time.
It is a perfume for the woman who has the instinct
to recognize a masterpiece at its inception.*

Compounded and Copyrighted by Coty, Inc. in U.S.A.

$000 • $50 • $25 • $15
plus tax

Coty

---

*I*n the early 1800s perfume bottles came with a secret compartment in which smelling salts were stored. Women wore tight corsets and were prone to fainting spells, so they needed to have a handy stash of smelling salts to revive them.

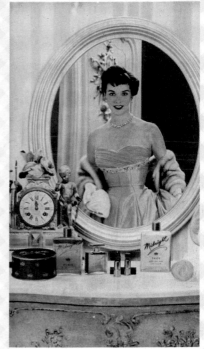

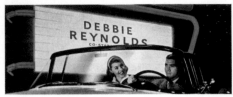

SHE: "I'd like to look just like Debbie Reynolds."

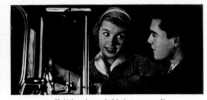

HE: "I think you're wonderful—just as you are!"

*To him
you're just as lovely
as a movie star*

He wants to be with *you*, rather than anyone else. So, to look your loveliest always, be sure you have a fresh glowing complexion like Debbie Reynolds. She uses daily new Lux care to keep it that way—and new Lux can do as much for you!

Cosmetic lather is the secret

New Lux lather has a beneficial cosmetic action on your complexion . . . actually helps your skin maintain the proper moisture balance. It's moisture balance, you know, that helps keep your complexion fresh, glowing.

For 15 seconds or so, gently massage Lux's rich creamy *cosmetic* lather into your skin. Rinse with warm, then cool water, and pat dry. That's new Lux care—the beauty care of 9 out of 10 Hollywood stars.

*New Lux is sealed
in Gold Foil*

. . . to protect its *cosmetic* lather, dazzling whiteness, wonderful fragrance. Only new Lux gives you both *cosmetic* lather and new Reynolds gold foil protection. Today you don't have to be a movie star to have a movie star's complexion—that's the beauty of new Lux in Gold Foil!

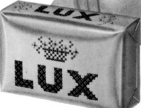

Debbie Reynolds

co-starring in MGM's

"THE CATERED AFFAIR"

a study conducted by the Smell and Taste Research Foundation in Chicago discovered that men find the smells of certain foods to be rather stimulating. The most effective scents for getting a physical reaction were combinations of lavender and pumpkin pie, doughnut and black licorice, and pumpkin pie and doughnut. Apparently a whiff of these grease-infused treats can harden body parts other than the arteries.

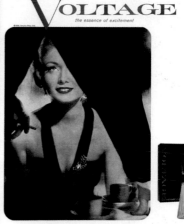

New and lavish
PINK CAMAY

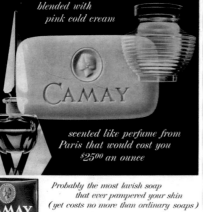

blended with pink cold cream

CAMAY

scented like perfume from Paris that would cost you $25.00 an ounce

Real Pink
CAMAY

Probably the most lavish soap that ever pampered your skin (yet costs no more than ordinary soaps)

Kept fresh and fragrant in Pink Pearl foil

I am your Avon Representative and I bring you fragrance news

Expect me with the new Persian Wood fragrance family... and a preview of Avon's exciting Christmas Gifts.

AVON cosmetics

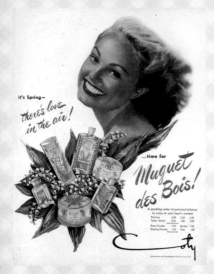

it's Spring—

there's love in the air!

...time for

Muguet des Bois!

A sparkling series of perfumed toiletries to enjoy to your heart's content

Perfume	3.00	2.00	1.00
Toilet Water	3.00	1.80	1.00
Face Powder	1.00		
Dusting Powder	1.25		

Coty

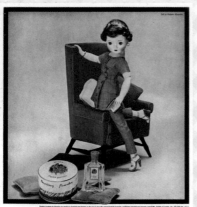

Gift or Madame Alexander

Makes you feel so fresh and feminine

Yardley English Lavender is unlike any other fragrance you've ever used. Because it's more than a lingering, lovely, lighthearted scent. It's a feeling . . . fresh, gay, wonderful—like being in love! And you know when you feel that good, you look your prettiest. Enjoy Yardley Lavender in many forms, give it with pride. You'll find it at your nearest cosmetic counter.

Yardley English Lavender toiletries, from $1.25. Dusting powder, $1.75. (Both plus tax.)

Yardley Lavender

"Just 30 extra seconds and I'm *Fragrantly Dainty* for hours"

"**HOW MANY GIRLS** realize, I wonder, how their popularity can be wrecked by body staleness? It took me months and months —lonely months—to learn *my* lesson. Now it takes me just 30 extra seconds to stay fragrantly dainty for hours. Watch:

"**FIRST,** I dry my body gently after my bath—just patting the places that might chafe."

"**NEXT,** I powder Cashmere Bouquet Talcum all over my whole body. Thirty extra seconds . . . yet it clings to me silky-soft as face powder and dries up any moisture I missed. There I stand, delicately perfumed all over . . . Now I know why you call it— *the fragrance men love!*"

"**NOW** my girdle—lingerie—stockings and frock. No chafing later; Cashmere Bouquet's silky feel stays on all evening. *And so does the fragrance men love*—to keep me fragrantly dainty for hours!"

Cashmere Bouquet is a body talcum of highest quality—the largest selling talcum powder in America. You'll love its haunting fragrance and clinging softness. Make alluring Cashmere Bouquet your daintiness secret. Available in 10¢ and larger sizes, at drug and toilet goods counters.

Cashmere Bouquet

THE TALC WITH THE FRAGRANCE MEN LOVE

134

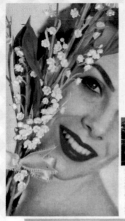

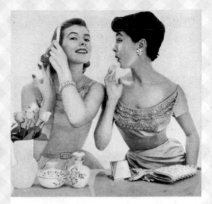
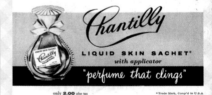
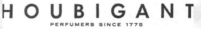
*W*omen and men's razors differ by more than just pastel colors and smaller size. Since the hair on a man's face is coarser than the hair on a woman's body, men's razors are at a much sharper angle.

135

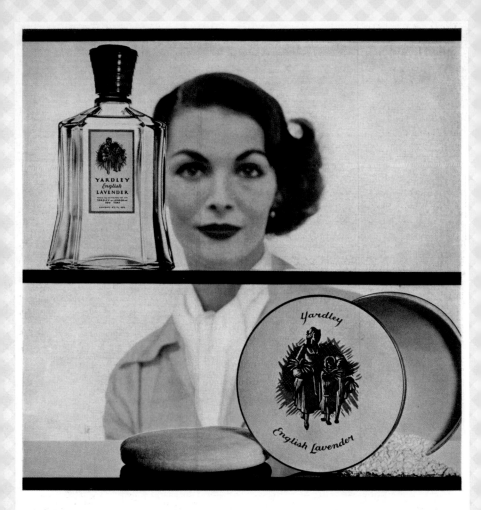

You look wonderful...because you feel wonderful

when you use

YARDLEY LAVENDER

for the freshest, youngest feeling in the world

It's so much more than a delightful essence. Yardley Lavender is a *feeling*. There's no lift like its crisp coolness, no other fragrance that makes you feel so fresh so long. Enjoy Yardley Lavender in its many other forms. The essence, from $1.10; dusting powder, $1.75 (all plus tax). Created in England, made in U.S.A. Yardley of London, Inc., 620 Fifth Avenue, N.Y.C.

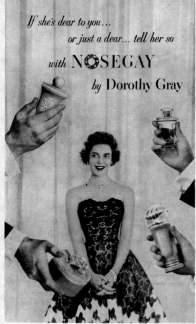

Bathe your way to Beauty!

BE LOVELIER ALL OF YOU!

A BIGGER CAMAY— JUST RIGHT FOR YOUR BATH!

CAMAY

COMPLEXION CARE FROM HEAD TO TOE!

CAMAY—SO PURE AND MILD!

MORE LUXURY— MORE LATHER!

FLOWER-LIKE FRAGRANCE TOO!

A Camay Beauty Bath gives all of your skin the finest kind of complexion care. Bathe every day with new Bath-Size Camay, and give your arms, your legs and your shoulders a true beauty treatment from head to heels. And you will rise from your bath clean and refreshed—just touched with the flower-like fragrance of Camay, the Soap of Beautiful Women.

CAMAY

Bath-Size Camay

for your CAMAY BEAUTY BATH!

*T*he "Twiggy" look was named after seventeen-year-old British model Leslie Hornby. She weighed about 90 lbs. soaking wet and inspired women everywhere to starve to try to reach her waiflike proportions.

If she's dear to you...

or just a dear... tell her so

with NOSEGAY

by Dorothy Gray

Miss Patricia Mullarkey, 1952 "Maid of Cotton," wears a dress of cotton lace over organdie by Celia Phillips.

The loveliest way to express what's in your heart is with Nosegay, by Dorothy Gray. This is the sentimental fragrance—young, but not gauche—tender, with a rare quality of making its wearer feel cherished.

What luxury!
Everything in Nosegay:
NEW HAND LOTION—4 oz....$1.00
DUSTING POWDER...$2.50
BUBBLING BATH SALTS...$2.00
EAU DE COLOGNE—4 oz....$2.50
EAU DE COLOGNE—2 oz....$1.50
Not illustrated
PERFUME—½ oz....$7.50
SOAP—3 cakes...$2.00
All prices plus tax.

wear NOSEGAY

by Dorothy Gray

America's *most loved* women do!

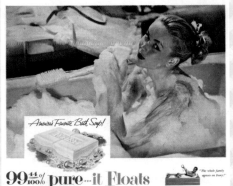

Howard Hughes used his
knowledge of airplane design
to construct the first under-wire bra
for Jane Russell to wear in the film
The Outlaw. Years later she became
a spokeswoman for Playtex's 18
hour bra.

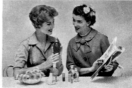

SPLASH and SPRAY
AVON FRAGRANCES...JUST HEAVENLY

Splash on Avon fragrance after the bath for the tingling sensation, for the luxurious way it wraps you in scent.

Spray on Avon fragrance after you've dressed, for the aura with which it surrounds you.

Your Avon Representative brings you a wide choice of scents to splash and spray. What fun you will have selecting fragrances that are just right for you!

"AVON CALLING" at your home to offer you an enchanting variety of fragrances to splash and spray.

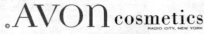

AVON cosmetics
RADIO CITY, NEW YORK

Now! There's Something

Thrillingly New!

in Palmolive's Famous "Beauty Lather"

New Fragrance! **New** Charm! **New** Allure!

And **Doctors** Prove Palmolive Can Bring You A Lovelier Complexion — Regardless of Age, Skin Type, or Previous Beauty Care!

PALMOLIVE

PALMOLIVE

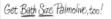

Get Bath Size Palmolive, too!

Use it in tub or shower.
The alluring new fragrance
of Palmolive's "Beauty Lather"
leaves you even lovelier *all over!*

Millions of women will prefer this "Beauty Lather" Palmolive over all other leading toilet soaps . . . the minute they try it!

And small wonder! For Palmolive's famous "Beauty Lather" has a new, clean, flower-fresh fragrance for new allure, new charm.

And using Palmolive Soap, the way doctors advised, is so effective that *all types of skin*—young, older, oily—respond to it quickly.

Dull, drab skin appears fresher and brighter . . . coarse-looking skin finer. Even tiny blemishes—

incipient blackheads—disappear or improve.

So do as Doctors advised. Stop improper cleansing! Instead, wash your face with Palmolive Soap three times each day, massaging Palmolive's wonderful "Beauty Lather" onto your skin, for sixty seconds each time, to get its full beautifying effect. Then rinse! That's all.

Yes, 36 doctors—leading skin specialists—advised this way for 1285 women, and *proved* Palmolive can bring lovelier complexions to 2 out of 3 in just 14 days. Get Palmolive Soap and start today!

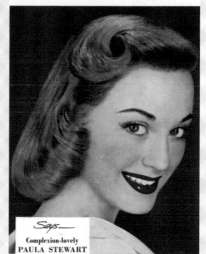

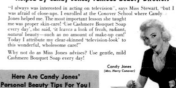
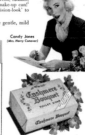

Chapter 5
The Feminine Finish
❖◆◇◈◆▣◈◇◆◈❖

As if it wasn't hard enough for women in the 1940s, 1950s, and 1960s to keep their hair lustrous, their skin glowing, their stockings run-free, and their lips and nails perfectly painted, women got a whole new set of unrealistic beauty ideals to emulate with the advent of color movies and the introduction of Hollywood as the mecca of glamour and celebrity. Not only were actresses larger than life, but so were their imperfections, including every magnified pore, follicle, and freckle on their noticeably pasty faces. In that era starlets suddenly realized that they needed even more weapons in their beauty arsenal to keep from fading into the woodwork. Classic beauty ideals were suddenly replaced with the need for camera-ready skin, and Technicolor friendly, photogenic features.

Flaws, both real and imagined, were broken down by body part. Bad breath or yellow teeth could doom one to social pariah status, while red scaly hands or chipped nails could stand in the way of a marriage proposal (who'd put a sparkler on those scraggly mitts?). To the rescue were products designed to depilate, smooth, soften, and if all else failed, cover up any imperfections.

Head to toe, women were faced with a new bout of insecurities. Mouthwash was "scientifically proven" to reduce bad breath and hinted at also providing a minty and robust social life. Products like Colgate dental cream promised not only fresher breath but also "Gardol," an invisible guard against tooth decay.

Women's bodies were on display like never before, with modest swimming costumes being rapidly replaced by bikinis and, in some radical cases, monokinis. Wayward body hair was public enemy number one. Companies like Lady Sunbeam and Remington Princess designed electric shavers in designer colors, encased in satin boxes resembling large jewelry boxes. As intense as this routine might have seemed during the bikini culture of the 1960s, these lucky women hadn't yet encountered our own generation's thong bathing suits and dare-to-bare Brazilian bikini waxes.

Handbooks instructed women on important accessories, including the proper gloves to wear with any and all "costumes" for both day and evening. As the century progressed, and salon services were no longer the exclusive domain of the very wealthy, women no longer regarded hats or gloves to be *de rigueur*, and they proudly displayed their fingernails.

Have the enlightened women of our own generation relaxed their self-imposed need for perfection? Not quite, but in many ways they've become more sophisticated in the pursuit of perfection, or at least in the methods by which they eradicate perceived imperfections. Teeth are whitened through the usage of everything from drugstore dental strips to pricy dental veneers. Tummies are tucked, furrowed brows are frozen smooth with Botox®, and unsightly bulges are massaged, rolled, or sucked out of bumpy thighs with liposuction. For many women, beauty has become a quest not only to beat the clock but also to completely erase the passing of time from their features.

Many women become their own worst critics, comparing their shapes and features with the buffed, polished, and airbrushed figures that grace magazine covers. Our increasingly narrow definition of what is beautiful leaves little room for individuality. In Hollywood the pursuit of manufactured perfection has spawned a surgically enhanced race of eerily identical lovelies with wraithlike figures, topped with bosoms of Amazonian proportions. Will our generation continue the tradition of worshiping only perfect icons? Ken Paulin, president of L.A. Promo, promotes dozens of new film releases each year and offers, "People become tired of individual celebrities but never the concept of celebrity." And so celebrities must keep evolving to meet glamour magazines' impossible ideals of perfection.

The French use the expression *jolie-laide*, which is a celebration of imperfection and is literally translated as pretty ugly. *Jolie-laide* reflects the fact that beauty comes in many shapes and forms, and just a hint of imperfection can enhance the beauty in anyone.

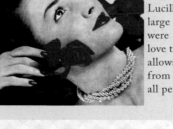

Classic and quirky beauties including Marilyn Monroe, Bette Davis, Barbra Streisand, and Lucille Ball came complete with full figures, large noses, bulging eyes, and shrill voices, but were beautiful nonetheless. We continue to love them most because their imperfect beauty allows us to believe that even though we are far from perfect by Hollywood standards, we are all perfectly beautiful in our own way.

BEAUTY CAN'T STAND SUCH DAILY ABUSE

Grave Risks to Teeth Found by Leading Research Clinic

See that cavity?

Brushing did it!

8 IN 10 ADULTS SUBJECT TO THIS INJURY!

*Recent studies at a leading Research Foundation clinic disclosed these startling facts:

OF ALL PATIENTS EXAMINED, REGULARLY BRUSHING TEETH WITH POPULAR DENTIFRICES, 58% ACTUALLY BRUSHED CAVITIES INTO SOFTER PARTS OF TEETH, EXPOSED BY RECEDING GUMS; THIS DAMAGE RESULTED FROM ABRASIVES IN THE DENTIFRICES; AND 8 IN 10 RUN THIS RISK CONSTANTLY.

—*(Reported in authoritative dental journal)*

NEW SAFE TEEL WAY—ONLY
One Extra Minute a Week!

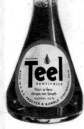

BRIGHTENS TEETH—*SAFELY!*

SEE the risk you may be taking with beauty! 8 in 10 may run that risk—says the report above!

Most adults have receded gums, exposing soft tooth structure that can't withstand abrasives in popular dentifrices. Gradually cavities are ground in. Then, ugly fillings.

TEEL—the modern liquid dentifrice—protects teeth because it cleans *without abrasives.*

And—note particularly—TEEL IS THE ONLY LEADING DENTIFRICE THAT CONTAINS NO ABRASIVES.

Start the scientific TEEL way now—before it's too late. And train your youngsters, too.

It's so simple! TEEL—*twice daily* —plus one extra minute a week spent brushing with TEEL and plain baking soda. This reveals sparkling beauty *fast*—and *safely!* Get TEEL today. There's beauty in every drop.

HERE'S ALL YOU DO

1. Brush your teeth every day — thoroughly — with TEEL. A few drops on dry or moistened brush. Feel it clean!

2. Once a week brush teeth with plain baking soda on brush moistened with TEEL. Brush at least an extra minute.

THIS NEW TEEL WAY CLEANS AND BRIGHTENS TEETH . . . LEAVES MOUTH DELIGHTFULLY CLEAN AND REFRESHED

TEEL COMES IN A BOTTLE — NO BOTHER WITH TUBES

Teel PROTECTS TEETH—*Beautifully!*

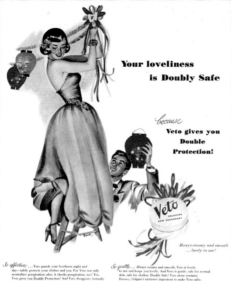

Your loveliness is Doubly Safe

because

Veto gives you **Double Protection!**

Always creamy and smooth ...lovely to use!

So effective... Veto guards your loveliness night and day—safely protects your clothes and you. For Veto not only neutralizes perspiration odor, it checks perspiration, too! Yes, Veto gives you Double Protection! And Veto disappears instantly to protect you from the moment you apply it!

So gentle... Always creamy and smooth, Veto is lovely to use and keeps you lovely. And Veto is gentle, safe for normal skin, safe for clothes. Doubly Safe! Veto alone contains *Duratex*, Colgate's exclusive ingredient to make Veto safer. Let Veto give your loveliness double protection!

Veto lasts and lasts from bath to bath!

$\mathcal{T}$he first self-made female millionaire in America was Madam C. J. Walker. The cosmetic entrepreneur was the child of former slaves, and developed products for African American hair and skin.

"Hey, Mr. Mennen— WHAT DO YOU MEAN—IT'S FOR MEN ONLY?"

ASKS **GUSSIE** *(LACY PANTS)* **MORAN**

Famous Woman Tennis Champion

"I like MENNEN Spray Deodorant better than any other deodorant I ever tried!"

"New Mennen Spray Deodorant has such a crisp, refreshing odor," says Gussie Moran. *"And it's wonderful the way it keeps away Perspiration Odor as long as three days with one application."*

CHECKS ODOR AND PERSPIRATION
Just Squeeze—IT SPRAYS!

MENNEN Spray Deodorant FOR MEN

59¢

• The spray deodorant made for men —and appropriated by women! • Quicker, much easier to apply! • Dries instantly, won't harm clothes! • Contains PERMATEC for longer-lasting protection! • You'll like its brisk, refreshing odor!

P.S. to the Ladies—Buy 2 Bottles One for Him...One for You!

145

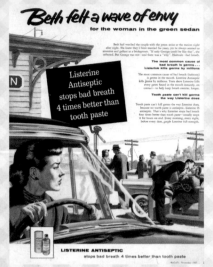
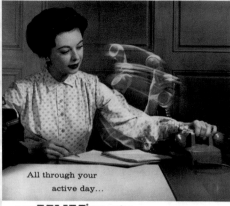

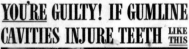
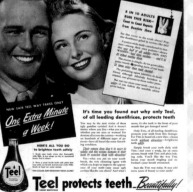

𝒯he earliest manicure might be the traces of henna found on the nails of mummified pharaohs.

𝒯he bikini is named after Bikini Atoll in the Marshall Islands, the site of early atomic testing. On July 11, 1946, Parisienne Micheline Bernardini was the first woman to model a daring two-piece.

Don't guess about your breath...

gargle LISTERINE and be sure

Anytime, anywhere, anybody can have bad breath, because most bad breath is caused by germs in mouth and throat. Listerine is antiseptic—to kill germs in mouth and throat on contact, by millions. It combines more active ingredients for killing mouth germs and stopping bad breath than any other leading oral antiseptic or mouthwash. Listerine stops bad breath instantly and for hours on end. *You actually feel it working.* **LISTERINE® ANTISEPTIC**

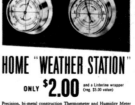

SPECIAL OFFER BY LISTERINE!

HOME "WEATHER STATION"
ONLY $2.00 and a Listerine wrapper
(reg. $5.00 value)

Precision, bi-metal construction Thermometer and Humidity Meter mounted on rich, wood-grained panel, for home or office.

ORDER NOW: Mail $2.00 (check or money order payable to Weather Station) your name and address, plus the wrapper from medium or large Listerine Antiseptic—to Weather Station, P.O. Box 292, Morris Plains, N. J. Offer good only in continental U.S., Alaska and Hawaii; except where regulated, licensed, taxed or otherwise prohibited by law. Delivery in 21 days. Offer expires August 31st, 1962.

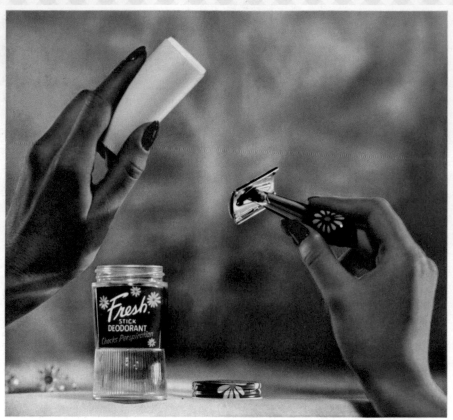

The one and only after-shaving (underarm) deodorant, and anti-perspirant

...And then Fresh Stick ! Imagine !

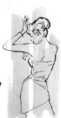

The anti-perspirant you can use any time...even after shaving.

Fresh scientists discovered it—the **new patented ingredient combination** that made all this possible. It's obtainable only in New Fresh Stick.

New Fresh Stick gets underarms dry, really dry, in seconds . . . **ends all danger of perspiration and odor.** And still it's safe for normal skin, no matter when or how often you use it. In addition, it's the only one that goes on dry, invisibly, without any greasy or runny messiness.

In New Fresh Stick you use this highly effective formula **full strength.** Yet, it's so gentle, so mild you can actually shave your underarms first and use it immediately afterward. Something most other anti-perspirant creams or sticks caution you against. But not New Fresh Stick. In fact, New Fresh Stick helps guard against after-shave infection because **it's actually antiseptic.**

Ever hear of anything like it? It's the newest—and greatest for daylong protection.

Fresh is a registered trademark of Pharma-Craft Corporation

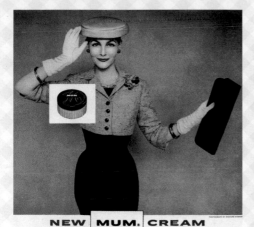

NEW **MUM** CREAM

**The doctor's deodorant discovery
that now safely stops odor 24 hours a day**

Underarm comparison tests made by doctors proved a deodorant without M-3 stopped odor only a few hours—while New Mum with M-3 stopped odor a full 24 hours!

You're serene. You're sure of yourself. You're handbox perfect from the skin out. And you stay that way night and day with New Mum Cream. Because New Mum now contains M-3 (hexachlorophene) which clings to your skin—keeps on stopping perspiration odor 24 hours a day. So safe you can use it daily—won't irritate normal skin or damage fabrics.

Another fine product of Bristol-Myers   Kind to your skin and clothes

---

*F*ormaldehyde, an ingredient used in the embalming of corpses, is a key ingredient of nail polish and nail hardeners.

*I*t took Carolyn Jones two hours to apply the makeup and two-foot-long human hair wig that transformed her into *The Addams Family* matriarch Morticia Frump Addams.

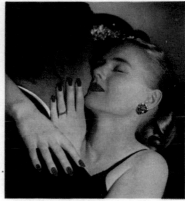

Now..."Home and You, dear"

Time for love and the deeply-desired softness of your hands. How do other women keep their hands welcomingly soft? "Young Marrieds" use Jergens Lotion, nearly 4 to 1; Jergens is, 7 to 1, the hand care of the Hollywood Stars.

Even more effective, now—thanks to wartime discoveries in skin-care. Jergens skin scientists can now make your Jergens Lotion even finer. Women made tests and said, "*Makes my hands even softer*"; and "*Protects longer*".

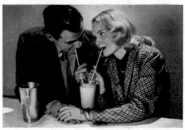

Dear familiar things—shared again. "*Sweet, your hands feel so soft!*" Two skin-softening ingredients many doctors use are still part of this even finer Jergens Lotion. In the stores now—same bottle—still 10¢ to $1.00 (plus tax). None of that oiliness; no sticky feeling.

For the Softest, Adorable Hands, use

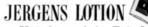

JERGENS LOTION

Now more Effective than ever—thanks to Wartime Research

149

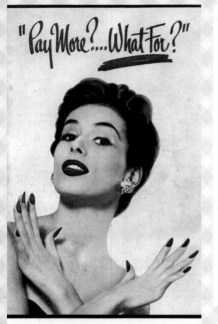

"Pay More?...What For?"

TESTS PROVE:

Even 60¢ nail polishes DO NOT out-wear

lovely, lasting CUTEX

IMPARTIAL TESTS by U.S. Testing Co. prove than even expensive 60¢ nail polishes do not out-wear, out-shine, out-glamour the fabulous new Chip-pruf formula brought to you by Cutex!

THE REASON—ENAMELON! Only Cutex, world's largest selling nail polish, contains this wonderful ingredient that prevents chipping and peeling. Keeps fingertips glamorous from manicure to manicure.

WHY PAY MORE? When Cutex gives you the loveliest, longest wearing colors—plus the safe Spillpruf bottle, not available in the 2 tested polishes. Discover Cutex today!

PREVENT BRITTLE NAILS . . . with gentle Cutex Remover. Contains not one drop of harsh, drying Acetone.

U.S. Testing Co. Report No. 66174, 11/18/53

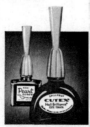

Cutex Nail Brilliance, 25¢
Pearl Cutex, 39¢. Prices plus tax.

Its cleaner, brighter *Taste* means cleaner, brighter teeth — *New Pepsodent* tooth paste with *Irium* removes the film that makes your teeth look dull!

Use Pepsodent Twice a day — see your dentist twice a year

The design for roll-on deodorant was inspired by a Biro ballpoint pen. Ban Roll-On was launched in 1952 and was packaged in a glass bottle with a large rolling ball top.

The first magazine dedicated to black beauty and grooming rituals, Ebony, debuted in 1965.

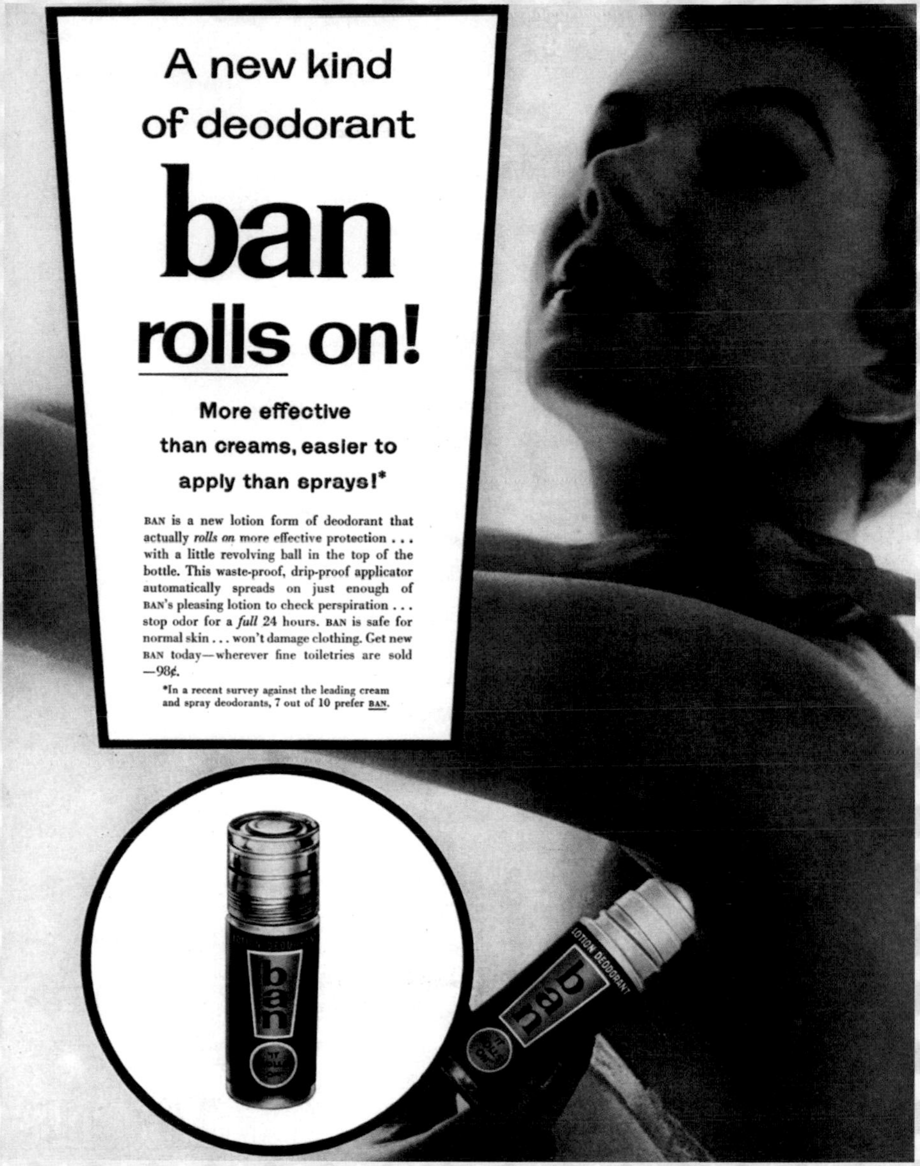
A new kind
of deodorant
ban
rolls on!
More effective
than creams, easier to
apply than sprays!*
BAN is a new lotion form of deodorant that actually *rolls on* more effective protection . . . with a little revolving ball in the top of the bottle. This waste-proof, drip-proof applicator automatically spreads on just enough of BAN's pleasing lotion to check perspiration . . . stop odor for a *full* 24 hours. BAN is safe for normal skin . . . won't damage clothing. Get new BAN today—wherever fine toiletries are sold —98¢.
*In a recent survey against the leading cream and spray deodorants, 7 out of 10 prefer BAN.
ban
LOTION DEODORANT
ban

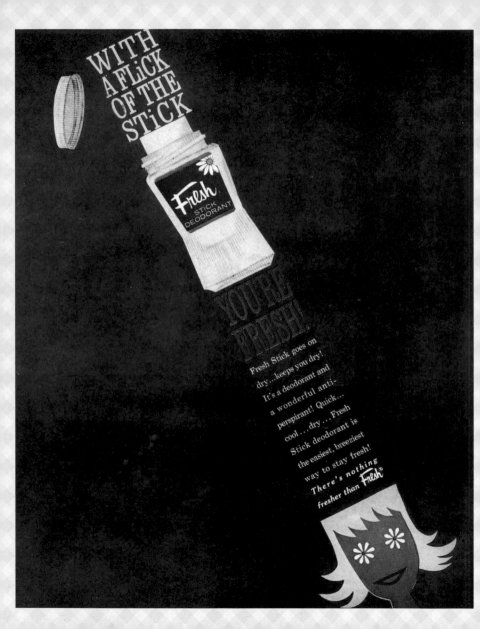

In Britain, skirts were taxed by length, which would account for the ever-rising hemlines. The invention of pantyhose and tights made the micro mini-skirt possible, since legs were still covered.

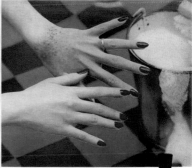

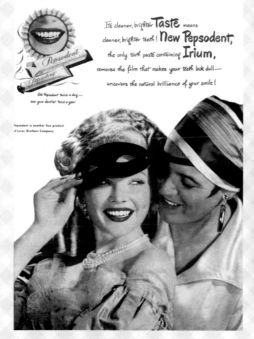

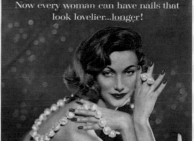
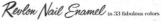

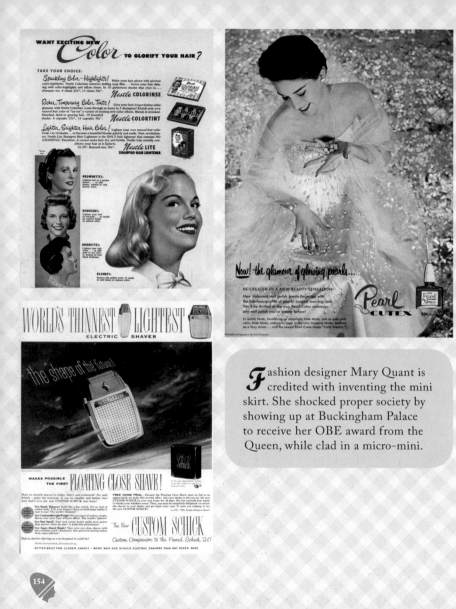

*F*ashion designer Mary Quant is credited with inventing the mini skirt. She shocked proper society by showing up at Buckingham Palace to receive her OBE award from the Queen, while clad in a micro-mini.

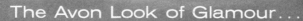

The Avon Look of Glamour...

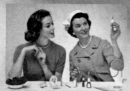

"AVON CALLING" at your home with new make-up ideas and other cosmetics and fragrances.

All eyes... lashes made lovelier with Curl 'n' Color, Avon's new and special automatic mascara; lids and brows beautified for total emphasis on the eyes.

Lips and fingertips twice lovely with new Twice Red . . . Add a touch of Fashion White Lipstick for the smart new moonlit effect.

Only your Avon Representative brings these make-up ideas to your home, for your personal selection.

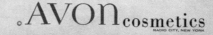

.AVON cosmetics
RADIO CITY, NEW YORK

AVON, CELEBRATING ITS 73rd ANNIVERSARY, IS DEDICATED TO BRINGING YOU THE WORLD'S FINEST COSMETICS

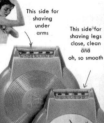
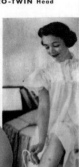

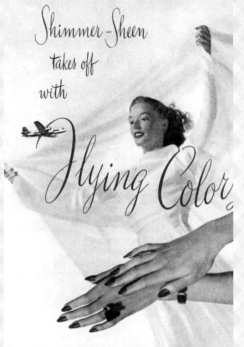

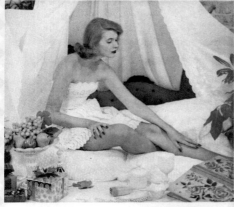

Important as your lipstick or perfume

At last, your personal grooming becomes easy ... quick ... actually fun! Once-over lightly with the trim little DUCHESS and your skin is smooth as a rose petal.

So fuss with soaps or creams ... no bothersome blade changing or chance of cuts. DUCHESS pairs so gently over sensitive underarm skin that deodorant may be applied immediately!

Better whisper in your personal Santa Claus about the new Remington shaver for ladies. (He knows its masculine counterpart ... the Remington 60 De Luxe. Probably made one himself!)

In fact, why don't you buy smart modern-girl cash other new Remington shaves this Christmas?

*Duchess Blue-or-Peppermint Pink, with slender matching cords, in a smart "jewel" case. A product of *Remington Rand*.

The Remington
Duchess
Electric Shaver

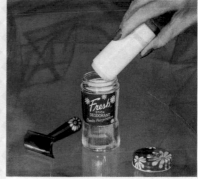
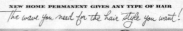
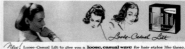
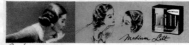
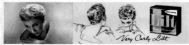
*P*arisian designer Andre Courreges's 1965 collection included white dresses worn well above the knee and paired with white mid-calf boots, spurring the Go-Go boot invasion. Nancy Sinatra's ode to this fashion frenzy, "These Boots Are Made for Walking," sold nearly 4 million copies.

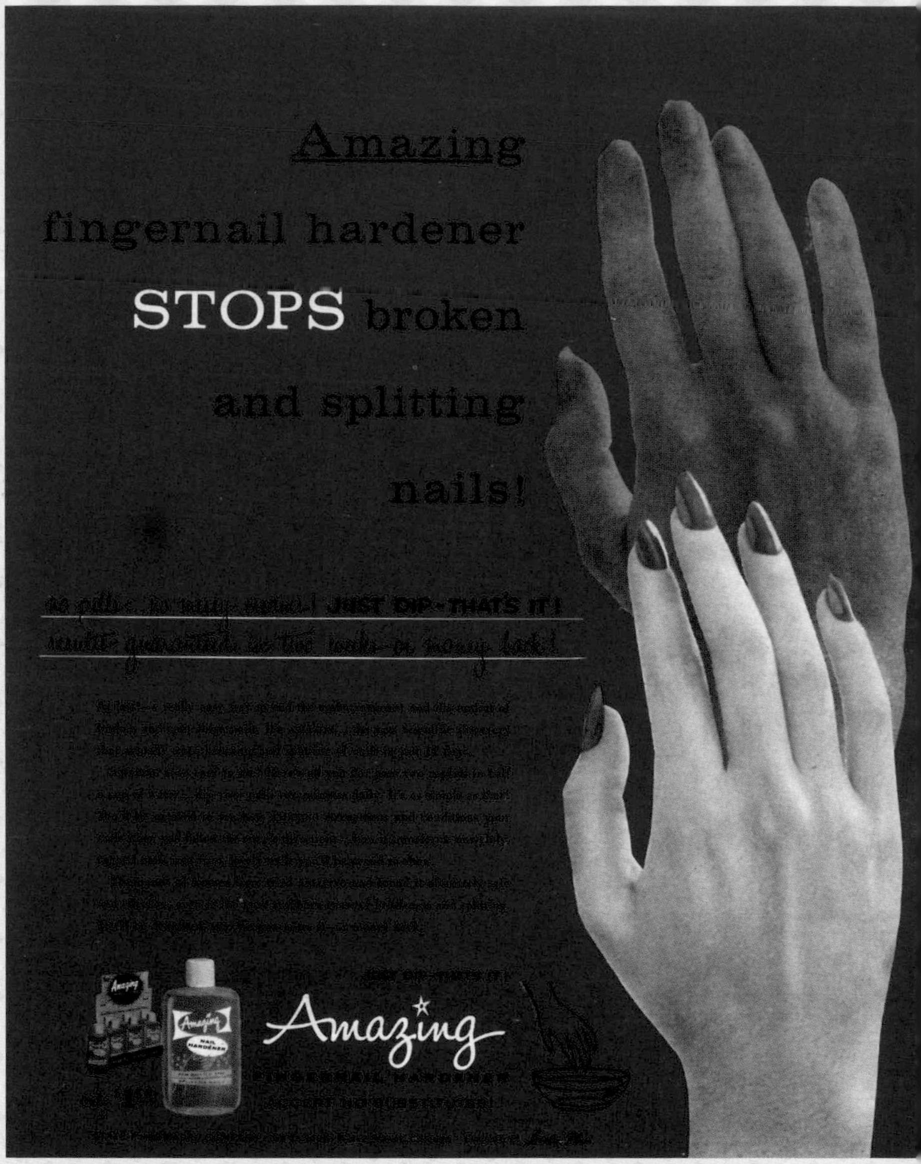
Amazing
fingernail hardener
STOPS broken
and splitting
nails!
JUST DIP—THAT'S IT!
Amazing
NAIL HARDENER

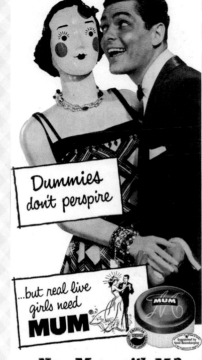

as important as your make-up...
your *Lady Schick*

Now... shaving even sensitive underarms
is so safe, so very gentle...you can shave as often as you should!

Like a great many other women, you probably feel you should shave more often to keep your underarms and legs always looking femininely smooth, feeling really clean. And what stops you? Chances are you're afraid of your blade razor . . . afraid of cutting and irritating your skin, especially under the arms.

Today, there's simply no need for that fear.

A *Lady Schick* Electric Shaver it so safe, so very gentle, you could shave every day if you wished! No nicks, no cuts, no painful irritation. *Lady Schick* is the one shaver with the "gentle-action" shaving head that's specifically designed for women. Easier to use . . . quicker . . . safe for even sensitive underarms.

So now, shave as often as you should...feel as feminine as you wish...choose a *Lady Schick!*

Lady Schick Electric Shavers . . . a perfect back-to-school gift!

*H*ollywood starlet Gila Golan spent her teens, with other World War II orphans, on a youth farm in Israel. She would do another girl's chores (including picking spinach) in exchange for the loan of a coveted pair of nylon stockings. (The beautiful girl who she borrowed these stockings from? My mother.)

Dummies don't perspire

...but real live girls need **MUM**

New Mum with M-3 kills odor bacteria ...stops odor all day long

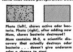

PROOF!
New Mum with M-3 destroys bacteria that cause perspiration odor.

Photo (left), shows active odor bacteria. Photo (right), after adding new Mum, shows bacteria destroyed! Mum contains M-3, a scientific discovery that actually destroys odor bacteria . . . doesn't give underarm odor a chance to start.

Amazingly effective protection from underarm perspiration odor—just use new Mum daily. So sure, so safe for normal skin. Safe for clothes. Gentle Mum is certified by the American Institute of Laundering. Won't rot or discolor even your finest fabrics.

No waste, no drying out. The *only* leading deodorant that contains no water to dry out or decrease its efficiency. Delicately fragrant new Mum is usable, *wonderful* right to the bottom of the jar. Get a jar today and stay nice to be near!

A Product of Bristol-Myers

159

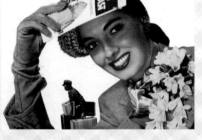
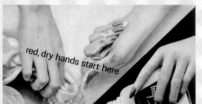
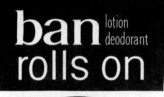
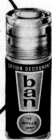

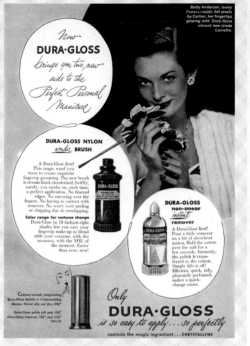

Christian Dior's "New Look" of 1949 included cinched waists, poufy skirts, and ornate detailing (some beaded evening gowns weighed close to sixty pounds). This supposedly "liberating" look practically hobbled women, who needed help getting dressed and getting in and out of cars.

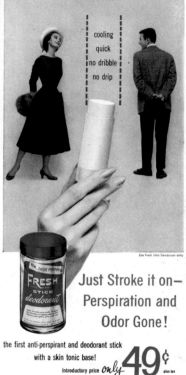

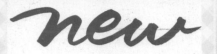

new

The first anti-perspirant deodorant stick with a skin-tonic base!

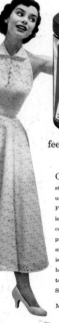

FRESH STICK deodorant

NOW...CHECKS PERSPIRATION

Apply to underarms daily. Closure, thumb-lift-on for lipstick, swivel-stick, leaves skin lightly glistening, fresh...

feels frosty... not waxy

Cool as snowflakes! Just stroke it on—odor gone, underarms *stay dry!* New Fresh Stick Deodorant is the refreshing way to complete deodorant protection. Special, effective anti-perspirant ingredient is blended with a skin-tonic base. So gentle, so pleasant to use . . . it's not waxy. Safe for fabrics. Use daily.

Memo to wives...buy one for him, too.

only 49¢ plus tax

FRESH STICK DEODORANT

keeps you Lovely to Love Always!

Fresh is a registered trademark of The Pharma-Craft Corporation.

*a*ccording to the Epsom Salt Council, during World War II cheap and affordable Epsom salts became popular for use in everything from skin softening soaks to homemade facials and foot baths. One of the earliest discoveries of magnesium sulfate, the scientific name for Epsom salt, occurred back in Shakespeare's day in Epsom, England.

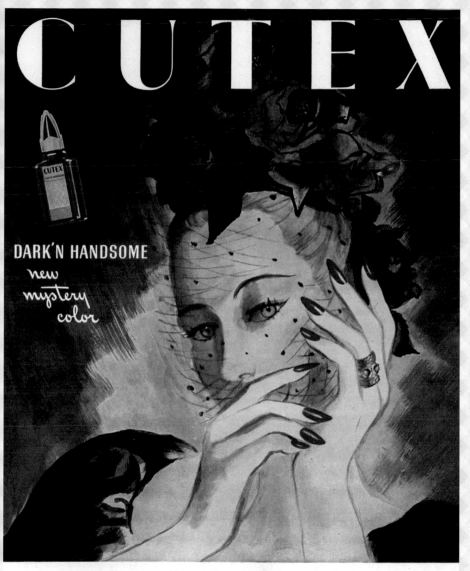

It's dark...it's exciting...it's the new Cutex color for intrigue. Put it on your long, temptress

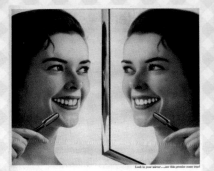

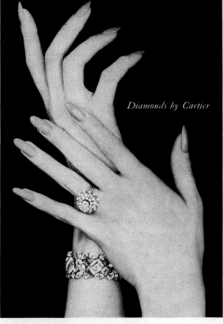
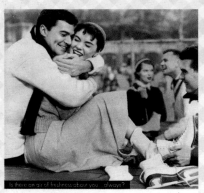
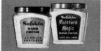
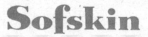

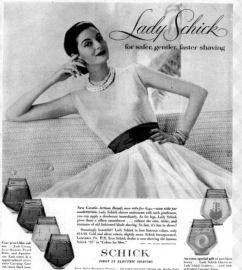
In 1955 Procter & Gamble introduced Crest, the first toothpaste with fluoride, which was proven to fight cavities and packaged in metal tubes rather than jars. One wonders what couples argued about in those days when squeezing or rolling the tube wasn't an option.

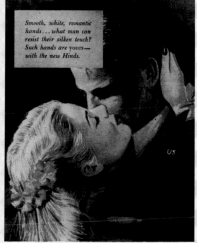
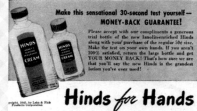

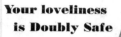

Your loveliness is Doubly Safe

because

Veto gives you Double Protection!

So effective . . . Veto guards your loveliness night and day—safely protects your clothes and you. For Veto not only neutralizes perspiration odor, it checks perspiration, too! Yes, Veto gives you Double Protection! And Veto disappears instantly to protect you from the moment you apply it!

So gentle . . . Always creamy and smooth, Veto is lovely to use and keeps you lovely. And Veto is gentle, safe for normal skin, safe for clothes. Doubly Safe! Veto alone contains *Duratex*, Colgate's exclusive ingredient to make Veto safer. Let Veto give your loveliness double protection!

Veto lasts and lasts from bath to bath!

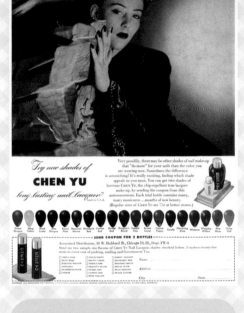

Try new shades of

CHEN YU

long lasting nail lacquer

Very possibly, there may be other shades of nail make-up that "do more" for your nails than the color you are wearing now. Sometimes the difference is astonishing! It's really exciting, finding which shade appeals to you most. You can get two shades of lustrous CHEN YU, the chip-repellent true lacquer make-up, by sending the coupon from this announcement. Each trial bottle contains many, many manicures . . . months of new beauty. (Regular sizes of CHEN YU are 75¢ at better stores.)

- - - SEND COUPON FOR 2 BOTTLES - - -

Associated Distributors, 30 W. Hubbard St., Chicago 10, Ill., Dept. FW-6

Send me two sample size flacons of CHEN YU Nail Lacquer, shades checked below. I enclose twenty-five cents to cover cost of packing, mailing and Government Tax.

Name
Address
City   State

*C*linique, introduced by Estée Lauder in 1967, was the first skincare brand that didn't base its image on glamour. Instead, Clinique touted itself as a functional and necessary part of a woman's daily routine—like brushing and flossing.

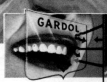
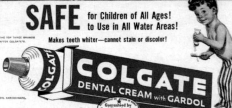

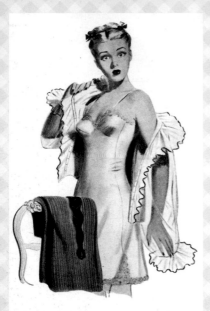

That blouse will catch more than the eye, Chick!

When underarm odor clings, men don't. So play safe with Mum

A stop sign for roving eyes—that froth of a blouse you're putting on.

Yet how quickly it can play false to your charm if it snags underarm odor. On guard, then, with Mum.

Your bath washes away *past* perspiration, yes. But you still need to hold onto that fresh start—to prevent risk of *future* underarm odor. That's why smart girls use Mum.

better because it's Safe

1. Safe for skin. No irritating crystals. Snow-white Mum is gentle, harmless to skin.

2. Safe for clothes. No harsh ingredients in Mum to rot or discolor fine fabrics.

3. Safe for charm. Mum gives sure protection against underarm odor all day or evening.

Mum is economical, too. Doesn't dry out in the jar—stays smooth and creamy. Quick, easy to use—even after you're dressed.

For Sanitary Napkins—Mum is gentle, safe, dependable . . . ideal for this use, too.

Mum

Product of Bristol Myers

Now Every Woman Wants

Lady Sunbeam

with the exclusive **MICRO-TWIN** Head

This side for shaving under arms

The other side for shaving legs close, clean and oh, so smooth

Enjoy new freedom from nicks, cuts and razor burns this safe, gentle, quick way

ONLY the Lady Sunbeam has a shaving head with one edge especially ground to shave the legs, and the other edge especially ground for underarm use. It is small as a compact. Ends muss and fuss, nicks and cuts of soap and blade. The Lady Sunbeam's gentle, sure performance gives you a new easy way to keep neat, fresh and dainty. Wonderful at home, or for travelling.

The modern electric way to feminine daintiness

Model LS in smart case $14.95.
Rich deluxe gift case, slightly higher.

Small as a compact —and fast, sure, convenient.

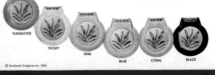

TURQUOISE   IVORY   PINK   BLUE   CORAL   BLACK

© Sunbeam Corporation, 1951

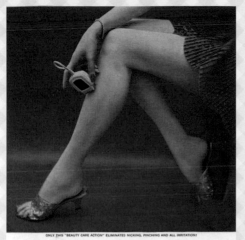

ONLY THIS "BEAUTY CARE ACTION" ELIMINATES NICKING, PINCHING AND ALL IRRITATION!

THE NEW REMINGTON PRINCESS ELECTRIC SHAVER
SHAVES RAZOR-CLOSE WITHOUT RAZOR-SCRAPE !

Once you try the new Remington Princess with "Beauty Care Action," you'll say goodbye to all old-fashioned "safety" razors and single-edge electrics.

For here is a shaver with not just 1, but 8 busy shaving edges, to stroke hair away completely, smoothly, quickly! Yet the Princess can't nick, scrape, pinch or pull your skin . . . thanks to Remington's exclusive Guard Comb!

A PRODUCT OF *Remington Rand*, ELECTRIC SHAVER DIV. OF SPERRY RAND CORP., BRIDGEPORT 2, CONN.

A shaving edges! Shaves back and forth. No switching sides for underarms and legs. Remington's exclusive Guard Comb protects skin from irritation.

In a lovely jewelry-type case . . . a perfect gift for Mother's Day.
PRINCESS PINK! $24.95 MAGNOLIA

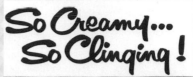

So Creamy... So Clinging !

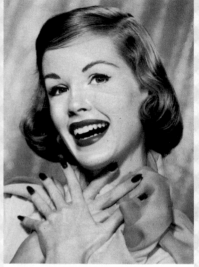

You'll be tickled pink!

Pink Cameo—Pink T.N.T.—Strike Me Pink— just three of the many sparkling springtime pinks created for you by Cutex! And if you like just the lightest "blush" of pink, try the new Cutex shade, "But Naturally"! One color is prettier than the next . . . all so feminine and flattering with the new fashions!

The creaminess your lips need—Cutex has it! It's the ONLY lipstick with creamy Sheer Lanolin. Protects against that dry, pinched feeling. Keeps lips smooth as a kiss!

The cling you want—Cutex has it! Color stays true and bright, even at night. Never leaves a kissprint! (Cutex makes Satin Cling Lipstick too! Ideal for girls who want 24-hour color with no drying after-effect.)

Why pay more?

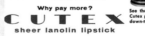

CUTEX
sheer lanolin lipstick

See the heavenly variety of Cutex pinks . . . all at such a down-to-earth price . . .
Lipstick, 69¢ and 35¢
Polish, 33¢ and 19¢

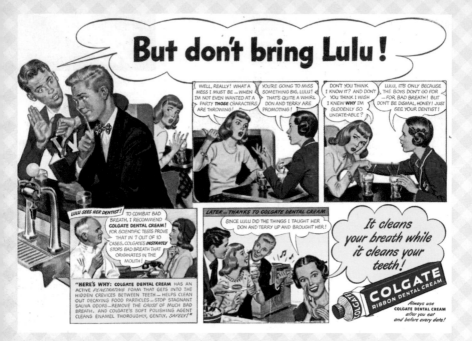

*M*etrosexuals might be a fairly new phenomenon that describes heterosexual men who take their hair care and grooming very seriously, but Elizabeth Arden introduced an entire line of men's facial creams and grooming products in the late 1950s.

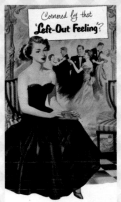
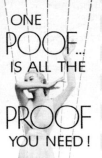
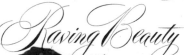
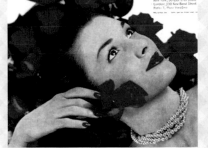

Now a <u>free dispenser</u>
for the gentle touch of Hinds

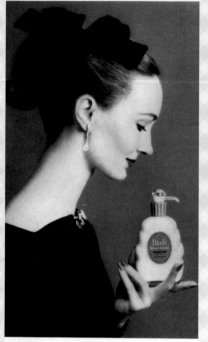

Now from the laboratories of McKesson comes the
first antibiotic deodorant
...used over 2 years by thousands of women to give longer, safer protection!

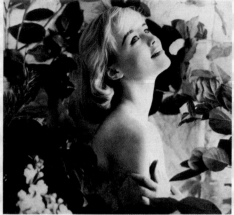

Fluffy, white Yodora won't irritate delicate skin. So mild, so gentle you could actually use it for underarm shaving.

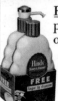

Fingertip dispenser free with purchase of two 49¢ bottles of Hinds Cream...all for 98¢

What a delightful way to pour on hand magic! Just press the new dispenser cap and Hinds special kindness will flow onto your hands. No spilling, no dripping, just the right amount. You'll love Hinds Honey & Almond Fragrance Cream. Like flowers, it contains a special ingredient, Floralex; puts a veil between you, wind, weather and work. Buy this offer now and get the fingertip dispenser *free*.

A product of Lehn & Fink • Also available in Canada.

AMONG the great medical discoveries in recent years is the use of antibiotics to wipe out bacteria.

Now, for the first time, an antibiotic is used to end perspiration odor. For what causes odor in perspiration, is the bacteria that breed there—and remain in your clothes, to make them objectionable too.

McKesson scientific research now ends this old problem with New antibiotic Yodora. New Yodora stops perspiration bacteria up to 48 hours. And gives this lasting protection without harsh chemicals so it does not injure clothing or irritate your skin. In fact, it is so mild and gentle that you could actually use this fluffy, white cream for underarm shaving.

It is only natural that McKesson laboratories, after years of dedicated research, should pioneer this amazing new principle to take care of unwelcome perspiration odor.

Ask your druggist, whose professional training you can trust, about New antibiotic Yodora. He can tell you why New Yodora is years ahead . . . why it does a better job, naturally to keep you and your clothes fresh and odor free. New antibiotic Yodora, in jars or tubes is economically priced. It is just another example of McKesson's great conscience for perfection, which always strives to "make it better—better for you." © 1957, McKesson & Robbins, Inc., N. Y.

NEW *
yodora
BETTER...by McKESSON

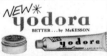

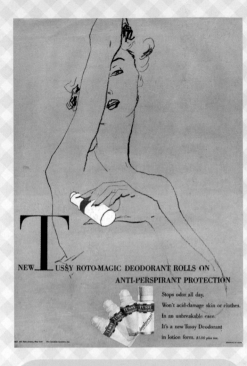

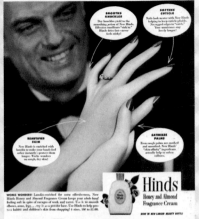

*I*n *I Dream of Jeannie*, Barbara
Eden was not allowed to show
her belly button because of the
unofficial "no navel" edict of network
television. It wasn't until years later
that Goldie Hawn bared her belly
button on *Laugh In*, as Cher did
on the *Sonny and Cher* show.

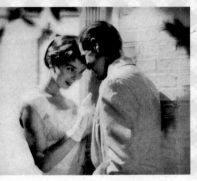

173

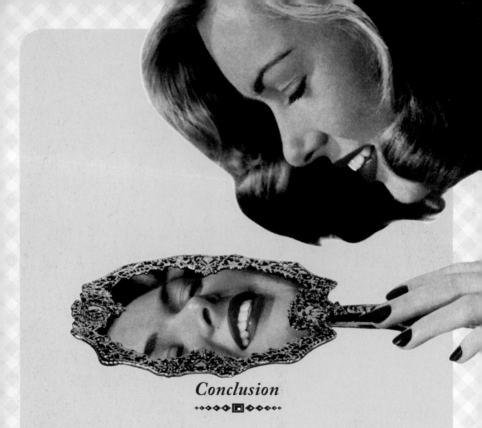

Conclusion

◈◈◈◈◇■◇◈◈◈◈

A half-century ago, the beauty industry was controlled by three tough broads on a mission of makeup and a desire to keep women looking younger for longer. Elizabeth Arden, Helena Rubenstein, and Estée Lauder fervently believed that their lotions, potions, and cosmetic devotion could take women to that beautiful place.

The multi-billion-dollar Lauder empire began in a modest kitchen in Queens, and Avon's humble origins have grown to $7.7 billion annually. Richard Murphy, a senior editor at *Fortune Small Business*, compares the cosmetic industry to the pharmaceutical and technology sectors, where major innovation is still contributed by smaller companies, though it's the behemoths with exclusive access to expansive marketing budgets that control the trade.

While specific wording may have changed, beauty exhortations haven't evolved that drastically in the past fifty years. In many ways what's old is new again—Estée Lauder's granddaughter Aerin is relaunching her own version of her grandmother's signature scent, "Youth Dew." Madison Avenue still relies on the reflected limelight of celebrities to sell product. Grooming rituals may have metamorphosed from beehives to Botox®, but the movies, literature, and icons of our own times are equally aspirational.

Literature has endlessly explored issues around the pursuit of beauty and the insecurity that often results. *The Second Sex*, the groundbreaking work of Simone de Beauvoir and the ode to imperfection of Helen Fielding, *Bridget Jones's Diary*, are just two examples from two different generations. Julia DeVillers, author of *Girlwise*, believes that teens bond with friends over the shared experiences of buying and applying makeup. AOL's Book Maven, Bethanne Kelly Patrick, said about the chick lit phenomenon, "Brand-names and beautification methods predominate. It's all about keeping things in check, be those things our hips, our jowls, or our deepest desires."

Musicians have also been using music to explore the notions of beauty for centuries. One such artist, esoteric musician Ben Lee challenges the concept of perfection or of one definitive beauty ideal. He refers instead to the Chinese Yin/Yang symbol of balance. "It contains dark and light, joy and sadness, gain and loss, high and low. Any time we get fixated on only one side of human experience, we are far from perfection."

At 6´4˝ tall, Rebecca Lobo of the WNBA doesn't fit traditional, narrow definitions of beauty. She believes that a beautiful woman is "sure of herself to the point that snide remarks or unfounded criticisms don't eat at her self esteem. In order to feel beautiful, women must have a confidence that has nothing to do with how they look."

In *West Side Story*, Maria famously sang, "I Feel Pretty." Her feelings about her looks were more important than actual physical beauty. She not only felt pretty, but also witty and bright (not to mention charming, stunning, and entrancing). At that moment of bliss and newly discovered love, it was the pure pleasure of feeling beautiful that made her beautiful. (Well, that and the fact that she was played by Natalie Wood.)

The secret then, to true beauty is finding the balance between looking beautiful and feeling beautiful, while enjoying the giddy, hopeful way that the tools of the trade can make us feel.

In other words, if you feel gorgeous, if you believe that you're gorgeous, you're already gorgeous!

Dedications

This book is dedicated to the everlasting chutzpah of Helena Rubenstein and Estée Lauder, two tough chicks who revolutionized the cosmetic industry and embodied the entrepreneurial spirit. And for everyone who has ever compared themselves to a beauty advertisement and thought they were somehow... lacking. Trust me, darlings, you're not. You're gorgeous, truly gorgeous.

Acknowledgments

I never realized just how many smart and supportive people I knew, until I started writing this book.

Many thanks to everyone at Collectors Press.

Big love to my family for always humoring (and mocking) me, particularly my mother, Judith, and sister, Kiki—two bombshells of our own era.

A lifetime of good karma to Allison Winn Scotch, and everlasting delicious inspiration to Bev Bennett, for being such wise and generous friends.

Hugs to Russell Barnett, Alex Gomez, Jeff McAdams, Amy Paturel, Ken Paulin, Erik Sherman, and Jill Evans.

Tons of gratitude to everyone who shared memories, anecdotes, and sources.